# ESSENTIAL OILS

FOR PROMOTING

# WEIGHT LOSS

# ESSENTIAL OILS

FOR PROMOTING

# WEIGHT LOSS

Speed Metabolism,
Manage Cravings,
and Boost Energy
Naturally

**SAMANTHA BOERNER**

PHOTOGRAPHY BY BIZ JONES

ROCKRIDGE PRESS

For general information on our other products and services or to obtain technical support, please contact our Customer Care Department within the United States at (866) 744-2665, or outside the United States at (510) 253-0500.

Rockridge Press publishes its books in a variety of electronic and print formats. Some content that appears in print may not be available in electronic books, and vice versa.

TRADEMARKS: Rockridge Press and the Rockridge Press logo are trademarks or registered trademarks of Callisto Media Inc. and/or its affiliates, in the United States and other countries, and may not be used without written permission. All other trademarks are the property of their respective owners. Rockridge Press is not associated with any product or vendor mentioned in this book.

Cover Design: Michael Patti
Interior Design: Jan Derevjanik
Art Producer: Maura Boland
Editor: Samantha Barbaro
Production Editor: Ashley Polikoff
Photography © 2019 Biz Jones.
Styling by Sophie Strangio
Author Photo courtesy of ©Angelic Jewel
Illustrations: © Shutterstock

ISBN: Print 978-1-64611-494-8
eBook 978-1-64611-495-5

R0

*To those who think you can't, you can.*

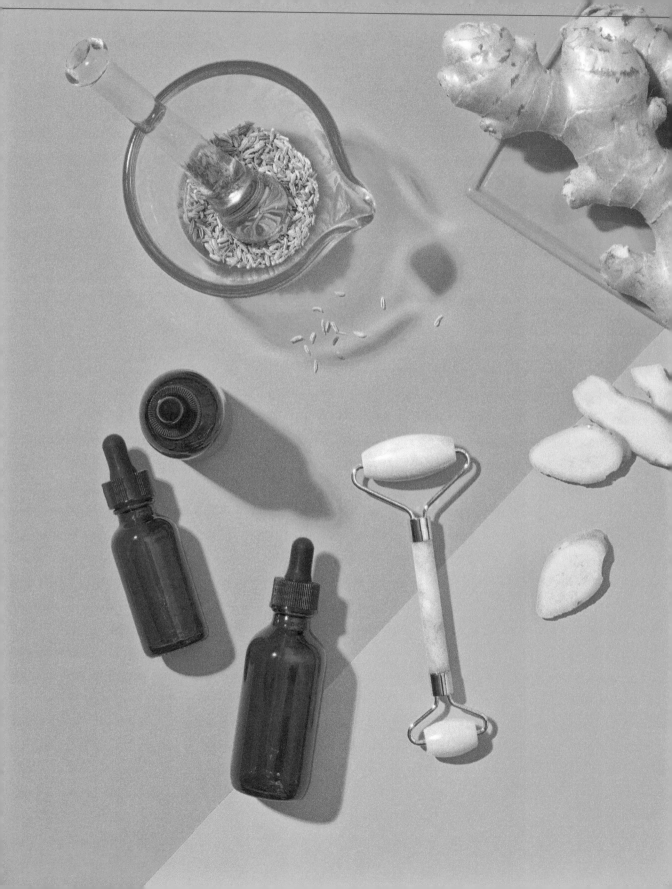

# contents

# introduction

Welcome, and I can't thank you enough for choosing this book! My name is Sammi Boerner, and I am honored to help you in your weight loss journey. I am the owner of Sage Mind and Body in Burnsville, Minnesota, where I offer custom aromatherapy, signature aromatherapy blends, and health and lifestyle coaching. I hold a NAHA Level 1 Aromatherapy Certification, Integrative Nutrition Health Coach Certification, and a bachelor's degree in Healthcare Administration from Liberty University. My goal is to assist you through your weight loss journey by providing you with essential oils and remedies to support your mind, body, and soul.

Since I was a teenager, I have struggled with anxiety, OCD, panic disorder, and insomnia. I was on three prescription medications and let those diagnoses control my life—until a little over two years ago when everything changed. I was overweight, unhealthy, frustrated, angry, anxious, depressed, and unhappy with my job.

I considered giving up, but then I started seeing a new chiropractor who helped me change the trajectory of my life.

It all started with a weight loss goal of five pounds, which I honestly didn't believe was possible. After just three months of eating clean and moving my body, I had lost 25 pounds. After six months, I had lost 50 pounds!

I had not thought it was possible to lose the weight and keep it off—and though I kept calling it a lifestyle change, everyone said it wouldn't last. My healthy lifestyle *has* lasted and, given how amazing I feel, I know I will never go back to where I was.

Along with the weight loss came a huge mentality adjustment. I am more positive than I have ever been and I feel fantastic, inside and out. I was even able to discontinue one medication for insomnia and have significantly decreased the dosage of my anxiety medications. It took a lot of dedication and belief in myself, which wasn't always easy.

Diet and exercise are crucial for losing weight, but they are not the only components of the process. I used essential oils throughout my whole journey to help with sleep, energy, anxiety, sore muscles, digestion, and to promote positive feelings and thoughts. I can't wait to share some of the essential oils that helped me in my journey, and I hope they help you just as much, if not more, than they helped me.

This book is broken down into two parts: In part 1, we'll review essential oil basics, methods of application, safety, and profiles of seven essential oils to help you through your own process of weight loss. Part 2 is full of blends and remedies for managing appetite, boosting metabolism, increasing energy, aiding detoxification, regulating digestion, improving sleep, and promoting calm.

I am so happy that you are taking this exciting next step. Weight loss can help you feel happier and healthier. I'm so excited for you to meet your goals and learn about your mind, body, and soul. You will quickly find out that you are stronger than you think you are—and when you meet your goals, you will look back at this journey and be incredibly proud of your accomplishments.

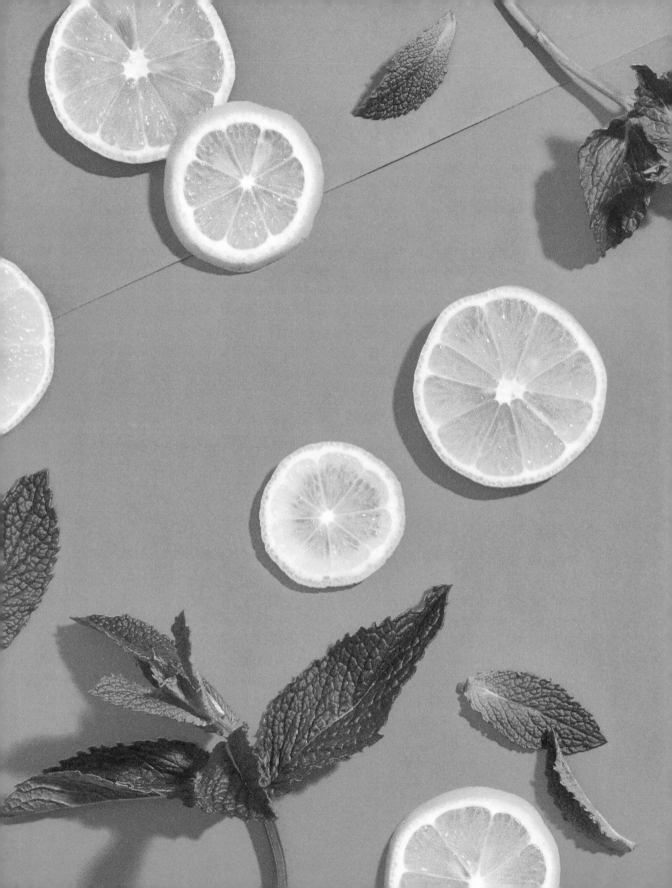

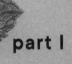

**part I**

# ESSENTIAL OILS & WEIGHT LOSS

In part 1, we will review the basics of essentials oils—including where they come from, how to use them safely, and different methods of application.

Essential oils help promote weight loss and balance in your life. We will review how essential oils can assist in boosting energy, managing appetite, increasing metabolism, reducing stress, improving sleep, promoting detoxification, and finding balance. Setting goals and achieving weight loss can be intimidating—essential oils will help you stay balanced, believe in yourself, and heal your body.

Think positive, stay calm, and keep moving forward.

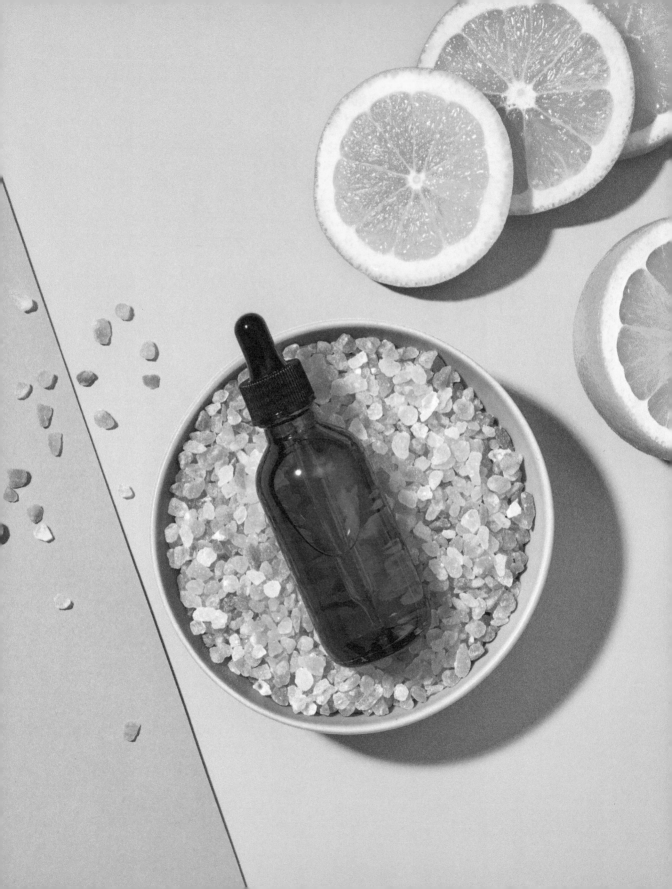

# essential oil basics & safety

This chapter will review the basics of essential oils, including what essential oils are, where they come from, how they are created, and how they are used. We will then go into general safety and types of application. Finally, you will learn how essential oils can assist you in your weight loss journey. When used correctly, essential oils can help you heal inside and out. Throughout this process, it is important to remember that you are in control and are capable of more than you know. Believe in—and be patient with—yourself.

# what are essential oils?

Essential oils are highly concentrated liquids created with aromatic plant material. Plant materials—such as flowers, woods, grasses, leaves, roots, resins, twigs, fruits, and needles—are harvested and put through either the process of distillation or expression (we'll get into the details of each one later) to produce essential oils. The number of essential oils is constantly growing, and researchers continue to learn more about which oils are useful as remedies.

The people of Mesopotamia used aromatic plants for religious and medicinal purposes (likely as far back as 5000 BCE), burning leaves, wood, and twigs for healing and protection. Ancient Egyptians extracted oils from plants to use in similar fashion, both for religious ceremonies and healing purposes. By the 18th century, aromatic plants, as well as balsams, wood, and resins, were being processed into essential oils more akin to what we know today.

Gradually, we learned about the astounding benefits and medicinal properties of certain aromatic plants through herbal medicine. Essential oils and aromatic plants were used to promote relaxation, induce spiritual awakenings and experiences, improve breathing, produce perfumes, create embalming fluids, heal burns and wounds, and reduce inflammation. They were even used to help fight the plague: The burning of aromatic plants around an infected area helped boost residents' immune systems and reduce the spread of the disease.

Each essential oil has its own chemical makeup based on how and where the plants were grown, how they were harvested, and whether the plant was distilled or expressed. We won't go into this too much, but it is important to know that this is where the therapeutic properties come from.

# where do essential oils come from?

Aromatic plant materials are harvested and put through the process of distillation and expression:

DISTILLATION is the most common process. It works with all types of plant materials and can be done with water, steam, or a combination of the two. Distillation occurs when plant material and water are heated to create steam and essential oil molecules. The steam rises above the tank into an outlet tube where it travels through a compressor and becomes a liquid. That liquid is then separated into a hydrosol and an essential oil. In this book, we will focus on and use essential oils, not hydrosols. However, it's useful to know that hydrosols are water soluble and are not as concentrated as essential oils. They are safer for internal use, as well as use on children, in gentle skincare products, in household cleaning products, and on rashes and wounds.

EXPRESSION, or cold pressing, is only used to produce citrus essential oils. When you squeeze an orange peel, you are expressing the plant material—meaning the essential oil molecules are being exposed. With expression, or cold pressing, the rind of the fruit is put under pressure to release its essential oils. Unlike distillation, heat is not part of this process and no hydrosol is created.

## Modern Essential Oils

Essential oils are becoming more popular, and research is helping us understand the true potential of these aromatic plants. Today, essential oils have numerous benefits and uses. Some health concerns that may benefit from essential oils are:

- ▶ Acne
- ▶ Anxiety
- ▶ Arthritis
- ▶ Chronic fatigue
- ▶ Constipation
- ▶ Depression
- ▶ Diarrhea
- ▶ Eczema
- ▶ Headaches
- ▶ Hormone imbalance
- ▶ Immune conditions
- ▶ Inflammation
- ▶ Insomnia
- ▶ Migraines
- ▶ PMS
- ▶ Psoriasis
- ▶ Respiratory problems
- ▶ Sinus infections
- ▶ Sluggish digestion
- ▶ Stress
- ▶ Thyroid disorders
- ▶ Weight gain

Essential oils are also great for beauty products, cleaning products, and personal care products. They can be used on their own or incorporated into things like body oils, cleansers, creams, facial oils, gels, salves, scrubs, and spritzers. And due to their high concentration, very little essential oil is needed to be effective.

I know what you are thinking: "How can a small bottle of essential oil cure these disorders?" It's important to clarify: *Essential oils do not cure or treat conditions*, but they are powerful products that can help reduce symptoms and create balance within the body.

In this book, we will focus specifically on how essential oils can promote weight loss. Essential oils do not *cause* weight loss, but they can help boost energy levels, manage appetite, spike metabolism, alleviate anxiety, improve sleep, promote detoxification and cleansing, and create balance in your body and your daily life.

## essential weight loss ingredients and equipment

Along with any weight loss equipment you already have in your home or at your disposal, you might want to stock up on these materials. This book has a variety of recipes to help you along your weight loss journey that include ingredients from the following list, as well as essential oils.

ALOE VERA GEL · We will use aloe vera gel to make Instant Energy Body Wash (page 69). It is a great way to start your day or to use pre- or post-workout if you are feeling sluggish.

BAKING SODA · If you prefer showers over baths, you will want to stock up on baking soda, as it is featured in the Deep Relax Shower Steamer (page 111) we'll make. I love using this relaxing shower steamer right before I go to

bed. It is a great way to unwind after a busy day.

CASTILE SOAP · Castile soap is another ingredient in the Instant Energy Body Wash (page 69). This is a great option for cleansing without having to worry about toxins in store-bought body washes.

CITRIC ACID · This can be found at most health foods stores and some major big-box stores. It is an important ingredient in the Deep Relax Shower Steamer (page 111).

EPSOM SALT · Epsom salt is a great tool in detoxification, flushing toxins, and reducing inflammation. We will use Epsom salts in a few recipes, including Detox Scrub (page 81), Purify Bath Salt (page 80), and Tension Relief Bath Salt (page 110).

PINK HIMALAYAN SALT · Pink Himalayan salt is great for clearing congestion, relieving muscle cramps and tension, and balancing the body's pH—it even has anti-aging properties. We will be using pink Himalayan salts in the Pre-Workout Salt Inhaler (page 61), Cleanse and Restore Bath Soak (page 79), and Soak Away the Day Bath Salt (page 109). It is very relaxing and great for promoting deep breathing.

UNSCENTED LOTION · The Stop Snacking Hand Cream (page 54) and Sore Muscle Relief Rub (page 67) will use an unscented lotion blended together with essential oils.

VEGETABLE GLYCERIN · This is an optional ingredient in our Instant Energy Body Wash (page 69). It will leave your skin feeling clean, refreshed, and moisturized. It's available at most health foods stores, but if you cannot find it, don't worry about it—the body wash will still be amazing without it.

## OTHER EQUIPMENT

DIFFUSER · Diffusers come in different types, shapes, and sizes. The recipes in this book will be for ultrasonic diffusers, which use water and essential oil to create a mist in the room.

FOAMING SOAP DISPENSER (12-OUNCE) · Make sure this is a plastic container. This will be stored in the shower, and we do not want glass to shatter on the floor.

PLASTIC PIPETTES · These come in different sizes and are ideal for measuring milliliters. You can find disposable plastic pipettes at craft shops and online. (For measuring quantities larger than 10 milliliters, a graduated cylinder may be more useful.)

GLASS DROPPER BOTTLES (2-OUNCE) · These bottles come with a lid that's also a glass eye dropper and are perfect for massage and body oils. Remember, you want dark bottles to protect the essential oils from sunlight.

GLASS EURO DROPPER BOTTLES (10-MILLILITER) · These are the bottles you see most essential oils stored in—instead of a glass eye dropper incorporated into the lid, they have an orifice reducer inserted into the neck of the bottle. The orifice reducer helps prevent the essential oil from oxidizing and makes for easy dispensing.

GLASS SPRAY BOTTLE (2-OUNCE) · Clear and Protect Spritzer (page 68) requires a glass bottle with a spray top. Again, make sure it's a dark bottle to protect your blend from exposure to sunlight.

INHALERS · An essential oil inhaler is a plastic tube with a cotton wick inside to absorb and hold the essential oils. Make sure you secure the cap tightly after each use.

LABELS · It is important to label each product you make. Write the name of the product as well as the ingredients used. If you won't be using all of the product soon after you make it, note the date on the label, too—remember that each ingredient in your blend has a different shelf life, so even an estimated "use by" date should be taken into account.

MASON JARS (8-OUNCE) · The bath salts and salt scrubs will be stored in Mason jars. The recipes in this book will yield eight ounces, but larger jars you may already have in your cupboard work just as well for storage.

PLASTIC SQUEEZE BOTTLES WITH FLIP TOP (2-OUNCE) · We will use these bottles for the creams and rubs we'll make.

ROLL-ON BOTTLES (10-MILLILITER) · These are great for on-the-go applications. It's best to get dark-colored bottles with a stainless-steel roller. The dark bottle will help protect the essential oils from the sun and the stainless-steel roller will provide smooth application.

## Storage

Proper essential oil storage is important to maximize shelf life and prevent oxidation. Oxidation occurs over time when essential oils are exposed to oxygen, causing them to break down. When these oils are oxidized, they can be irritating to the skin and are more likely to cause allergic reactions. Exposure to sunlight can cause similar degradation. Here are some tips and tricks for storing your essential oils:

▸ Essential oils should be stored in dark glass bottles. The dark color protects the essential oil from sunlight. The most common colors you're likely to find in stores are amber and cobalt, but other dark colors will work. Bottles should never be stored in direct sunlight.

▸ If you are blending essential oils with other products, glass containers are preferred. BPA-free plastic will work if that is all that is available.

▸ Keep essential oils in a cool, dark place, especially if they are citrus oils. Citrus oils oxidize faster and can cause skin irritations when oxidized. For best results, citrus oils should be refrigerated.

▸ Tightly secure bottle caps after each use to prevent oxidation.

▸ Essential oil bottles should have an orifice reducer cap to keep as much oxygen out of the bottle as possible. This also makes it easier to dispense the oil.

## Carrier Oils

Carrier oils are important ingredients in essential oil recipes for a few reasons. These carrier oils (which are vegetable, nut, and seed oils) aid in optimal absorption of essential oils. Diluting strong essential oils with carrier oils also helps reduce potential skin reactions. Plus, carrier oils have oil-soluble vitamins (including vitamins A, D, and E) and essential fatty acids, which are great for maintaining healthy skin tone, texture, and strength. Here are five popular carrier oils and each of their benefits:

ALMOND OIL is great for all skin types. It protects, softens, soothes, and nourishes the skin. It helps with healing wounds and cuts, softening and toning the skin, reducing age spots, reducing inflammation, fading scars, and even reversing sun damage. Almond oil is absorbed into the skin very quickly, but it can leave an oily feeling after application. It is a pale yellow color, has very little to no aroma, and is gentle enough to be used as a facial or body oil.

AVOCADO OIL works best with sensitive, dry, and mature or fragile skin.

Since it is high in antioxidants, it has powerful anti-aging effects. It is also beneficial for hydrating, soothing, tightening, and reducing inflammation. Its anti-inflammatory properties make avocado oil helpful in treating skin conditions such as acne, eczema, and psoriasis. It is easily absorbed into the skin and provides a protective barrier. The oil has a pale yellow color and a very mild aroma.

COCONUT OIL is great for dry and damaged skin. It is white and much thicker than other carrier oils. Similar to avocado oil, it is high in antioxidants and therefore has anti-aging benefits. It has a light feeling and absorbs into the skin well without leaving you feeling greasy. If you have acne-prone skin, avoid using coconut oil daily as it can block pores and cause blemishes. It doesn't always cause blemishes, though, so don't be afraid of using it! It is extremely moisturizing and softens the skin instantly.

JOJOBA OIL can be used on all skin types and works best for acne, combination, and oily skin as it clears clogged pores. It is a very light oil, yellow in color, and odorless. Jojoba oil is extremely hydrating without leaving the skin greasy. This gentle oil helps reduce the appearance of scars, wrinkles, and stretch marks. It is high in vitamin E

and therefore great for soothing burns and healing wounds.

SESAME OIL is heavier than the other oils listed here. It penetrates the skin and then travels deeper into the tissue. This oil is great for skin conditions like arthritis, eczema, and psoriasis, as well as muscle aches and pains, as it is soothing, gentle, and anti-inflammatory. Due to its antibacterial and antiviral properties, sesame oil is also great for treating skin infections such as acne, athlete's foot, and shingles. It improves circulation in the body, helping reduce the appearance of cellulite. It is dark yellow in color and has a strong smell.

# safety & dilution

Because of the high concentration of aromatic plant material, exercising safety with essential oils is very important. Here are some general safety recommendations:

▸ Dilution is extremely important. We're often trained to believe that more is better, right? I learned the hard way—you need to learn about proper dilution before using essential oils. Not diluting essential oils properly can result in irritation of skin or mucous membranes, allergic reactions, permanent sensitivity, and photosensitization (sensitivity to sunlight). When essential oils are diluted, they are more effective as well as more cost-effective. ***Never apply essential oils to the skin undiluted.***

▸ It is important to know the quality of the essential oils being used. How were the aromatic plants grown and harvested? You want to make sure you are getting a product that is organic, wild harvested, or unsprayed. Look into the products before purchasing, and don't just rely on the bottle's label using terms like therapeutic, professional, or medical grade.

▸ Essential oils should *never* come in contact with the eyes. Make sure to wash your hands after applying essential oils.

▸ Stay out of the sun or tanning booths for at least 12 hours after using a photosensitizing essential oil. These cause discoloring and burning of the skin when exposed to ultraviolet rays. I have noted the blends in this book that use photosensitizing oils (grapefruit and lemon), but when you're going beyond these recipes it's important to learn which essential oils fall into this category.

▸ Avoid using the same essential oil for a long period of time to avoid sensitization.

▸ Keep essential oils out of the reach of children.

## DILUTION GUIDE

| | 0.5% dilution | 1% dilution | 2% dilution | 3% dilution | 4% dilution | 5% dilution |
|---|---|---|---|---|---|---|
| **5 ml = 1 tsp = ⅙ oz** | | 1 drop | 2 drops | 3 drops | 4 drops | 6 drops |
| **10 ml = 2 tsp = ⅓ oz** | 1 drop | 2 drops | 4 drops | 6 drops | 8 drops | 12 drops |
| **15 ml = 3 tsp = ½ oz** | 2 drops | 3 drops | 6 drops | 9 drops | 12 drops | 18 drops |
| **30 ml = 6 tsp = 1 oz** | 4 drops | 6 drops | 12 drops | 18 drops | 24 drops | 36 drops |
| **60 ml = 12 tsp = 2 oz** | 8 drops | 12 drops | 24 drops | 36 drops | 48 drops | 72 drops |
| **120 ml = 24 tsp = 4 oz** | 16 drops | 24 drops | 48 drops | 72 drops | 96 drops | 144 drops |

## Cautionary Oils and Vulnerable Populations

It is important to consult a physician or certified aromatherapist before using essential oils on infants and pets or during pregnancy, due to the potency of the aromatic plant material. Use extreme caution when using essential oils on children and seniors. Some essential oils can be irritating to the skin even when they are diluted. Always read labels and instructions before using—when in doubt, do not use.

## Combining Oils Safely

When creating essential oil products, always blend the essential oils first and then add them to the product base (carrier oil, lotion, or gel). This will allow the essential oils to blend together properly. Combining essential oils is generally safe, but it is important to make sure you are diluting them properly before using them topically.

# safe dosage & application

The dosage of essential oils varies based on what products you are creating and the type of application. Here are some general dilution guides that will be followed in the recipes throughout this book.

**0.5% DILUTION** is best for elderly individuals or individuals with thin or sensitive skin.

**1% DILUTION** is best for facial gels and creams, as well as for use with children and pregnant women.

**2% TO 4% DILUTION** is the most common dilution rate. It is used for massage oils, body oils, facial oils, creams, lotions, and general skincare. The dilution rate will vary between 2% and 4% depending on what the goals are with the product.

**5% DILUTION** is used for localized treatments, salves, wounds, and muscle aches and pains.

**10% DILUTION** can be used for muscular aches and pains or acute pain. However, 10% dilution should only be used occasionally for acute pain as it can cause skin sensitization.

## Skin Application

Essential oils can be used topically when diluted or when blended into a product base such as a carrier oil, gel, water, or salve. Topical use of essential oils is best for helping with concerns such as anxiety, burns, circulation, depression, fatigue, headaches, weakened immunity, inflammation, insomnia, joint pain, migraines, muscle pain and tension, skin issues, sprains, stress, and varicose veins. Essential oils can be incorporated into body oils, cleansers, toners, bath salts, scrubs, gels, and salves.

The skin has three main layers that absorb the oils and direct them into the body for healing. One of the most effective places to apply essential oils is on the bottoms of your feet. Your feet have large pores that can easily absorb products, and the skin is less sensitive. In reflexology, every part of the bottoms of your feet are connected to an organ. (For example, your big toe is connected to the brain, pineal gland, and pituitary gland.)

When using essential oil products topically, it is important to perform a patch test before use. To patch test, take a small amount of product and apply it to your forearm. Wait 24 hours and if no reaction occurs, proceed with normal product use. If any reaction occurs, discontinue use immediately and follow up with a physician. Patch testing is important, even when using diluted essential oils or using products containing essential oils such as lotions, gels, massage oils, or facial oils.

## Inhalation

Inhalation is the act of breathing in an aromatic substance. It is known best for helping with issues like anxiety, depression, headaches, insomnia, migraines, nausea, respiratory issues, and stress. Inhalation can be done through diffusion, directly from the bottle, directly from the palms of your hands, or through salt inhalers and steams. Diffusion disperses the essential oil molecules into the air—certain oils can even disinfect the air. Inhalation direct from the bottle, direct from the palms of your hands, or from an inhaler is best for times of emotional distress and meditation that focuses on deep breathing. Inhalers are also great for on-the-go use as they are small and compact, yet effective. Smelling salt inhalers and steams with essential oils are great for respiratory concerns such as congestion, sinus infections, and respiratory infections.

## Ingestion

The amount of plant material in one drop of essential oil is very high. Some essential oils when taken internally can be toxic. It takes years of training to learn about safe internal use, so please consult an aromatherapist who specializes in internal use before ingesting any essential oils. *Even if the bottle says it is safe for internal use, it's still important to consult your physician or aromatherapist before doing so.* We will not ask you to ingest any essential oils in this book.

Used safely and properly, essential oils and aromatherapy follow a holistic approach to create balance in our bodies. The more balanced we are mentally and physically, the more likely our bodies will be receptive to weight loss. The journey isn't always easy, but in the end you will feel more happy, confident, and strong.

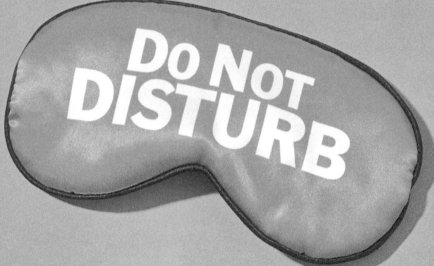
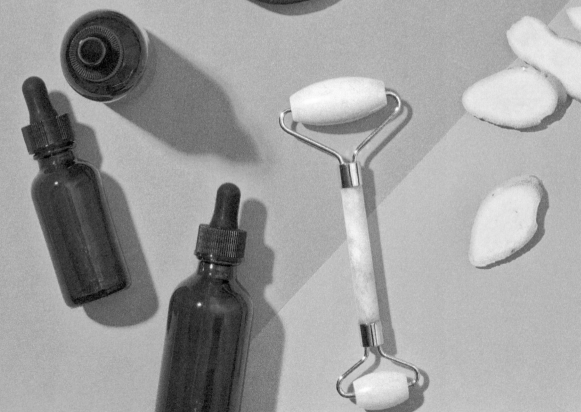

# promoting weight loss with essential oils

Essential oils are tools for helping you bust through any roadblocks that may arise. If you feel tired, hungry, crabby, sluggish, angry, frustrated, or constipated, or even if you just don't feel comfortable in your own skin, essential oils can help! They are invaluable tools you will want by your side throughout this journey.

# how can essential oils help with weight loss?

Have you felt like you are doing everything right, but you still aren't losing the weight? Have you hit a plateau? Did you lose the ambition you had when you started?

Essential oils can help you with the following:

▸ Boost your energy so you don't constantly feel tired

▸ Boost your metabolism to burn calories and promote weight loss

▸ Calm anxiety

▸ Clear your mind so you can focus on your goals

▸ Create balance in your daily life

▸ Create balance in your body

▸ Curb cravings so you don't feel the need for sweet or salty foods

▸ Encourage detoxification so you can rid your body of impurities and toxins

▸ Give you an energy boost pre-workout so you can reach your full potential

▸ Improve the texture, elasticity, and tone of your skin

▸ Increase energy in the morning so you can start your day off right

▸ Push through challenges you might face during your weight loss journey

▸ Reduce inflammation in the body to reduce joint pain

▸ Reduce inflammation in the gut so you don't feel bloated and puffy

▸ Regulate digestion so your body can eliminate properly

▸ Relieve sore muscles pre- and post-workout

▸ Relieve stress

▸ Promote relaxation so you can sleep deeply and wake refreshed

▸ Suppress your appetite so you aren't overeating or snacking

The possibilities are nearly unlimited!

Losing weight can be stressful, and merely thinking about the process can be daunting. People tend to focus on the results and want to skip ahead to the end. Unfortunately, that isn't possible. What *is* possible? Setting goals, believing in yourself, and going with the flow. It isn't always easy to let go of control, but if you can trust the process, you'll learn so much about yourself and your body. You are stronger than you think you are! When you reach your goals, you will look back and be proud of yourself.

Just two years ago, I was 40 pounds heavier, unhappy with my life, uncomfortable with my body, frustrated, sad, and anxious—and felt I was alone. I had people around me, but I couldn't let others love me because I didn't love myself.

One day, I decided something needed to change. I started seeing a chiropractor who worked with me on a cleanse, and I gradually changed to a plant-based diet. Throughout this journey, I used essential oils every day—to energize, aid digestion, promote detoxification, increase confidence, clear my mind, reduce inflammation, and decrease anxiety. Essential oils have been a huge part of my weight loss journey, and I can't wait to share recipes to help you along your own journey.

## ALONG WITH DIET AND EXERCISE . . .

While essential oils assist in achieving weight loss goals, they won't work by themselves. Diet and exercise are crucial, and it is important to understand neither are one size fits all.

For example, I follow a vegan, gluten-free diet and mostly avoid artificial sugar, but that is not for everyone. Hundreds, if not thousands, of diets have been created over the years, so it may take time to find what works best for you. The same goes with exercise. One person might do HIIT workouts daily while another person's body can't handle HIIT every day. You will need to experiment and find what works best for you, your lifestyle, and your body.

When you put the time and effort into changing your diet and exercise, you will see results. There isn't a guaranteed timeline or a magic potion that will cause weight loss or cure you of all ailments. Take your time and be patient with yourself. The change is deep within you. Find that fire within you, set realistic goals, make small adjustments to your diet, exercise, try different blends from this book, and always remember to believe in yourself. You can do it!

## Other Factors

Diet and exercise are not the only factors in promoting weight loss:

▸ Are you drinking alcohol? Alcohol is high in calories and can add up quickly. Decrease alcohol intake as much as possible so you can see results and reduce inflammation in your body.

▸ Are you drinking plenty of water? Try drinking half your body weight in ounces (for example, if you weigh 160 pounds, drink 80 ounces or 10 cups a day). If you are exercising or drinking sugary beverages, you will need to increase your water intake. Being hydrated is key when going through a diet or detox.

▸ Are you getting enough sleep? Is it good quality sleep? The quality of your sleep can set the tone for the day. When you sleep well, you can be more energized, motivated, positive, and goal-oriented.

▸ Are your goals and expectations realistic? Goal-setting is extremely important—but if the goals you set are too high, you are more likely to get frustrated and less likely to progress. Start small and as you make progress, re-assess your goals.

▸ Do you eat clean but still drink beverages high in sugar? Sugar causes inflammation and turns into fat. It also spikes your blood sugar levels, which can make you fatigued and hungry.

▸ Do you have a medical or genetic condition? This may play a role in weight gain and weight loss. Check in with your physician if you feel this might be a concern.

▸ Do you have ways to relieve and manage stress in your daily life? Stress puts your body in the fight-or-flight response, and in this state your body doesn't have time to rest and digest. Stress can also cause inflammation and chronic illness.

▸ Do you think your hard work isn't paying off because the scale shows a higher number than before? Sometimes weight alone isn't a helpful measurement—muscle weighs more than fat, so when you're gaining muscle from exercise you may actually weigh more. Look for "non-scale" victories. Do your clothes fit better? Instead of looking at the scale, taking measurements is very helpful in knowing how your body is responding.

▸ What products are you putting on your skin? Your skin is your largest organ, as well as the protective layer for the other organs. Make sure you are using products with as few ingredients and as pure as possible.

# a holistic approach

Aromatherapy follows a holistic approach to create balance within the mind, body, and soul. A holistic approach looks at the whole person, as well as their environment, stress levels, family life, work life, and other social factors. One of the goals of this book is to provide you with essential oil blends and products that will promote physical, mental, and emotional well-being. I want to help you find what works best for you and your body so you can feel happy and healthy as well as reach your goals. Who doesn't want to feel balanced? Life happens and problems inevitably arise. But the more balanced you are, the better you can handle life and all of the challenges that come your way.

## Essential Oils Can Boost Energy

If you ask someone how they are, they will probably say they are tired or busy. Everyone is constantly on the go, and it's no surprise if you can't find the time necessary to recharge.

You might be getting adequate amounts of sleep and still feel lethargic. You might unknowingly be following the wrong diet and so you're not getting enough nutrients. Maybe you aren't working out because of how tired you are, or perhaps you're very worn-out after workouts. Maybe technology is draining you. Or maybe you had energy before you started changing your diet and exercise routine. It is normal during times of change to feel low on energy, and it is hard to go through your day with low energy.

Some essential oils naturally boost your energy and motivation. They can be used right away in the morning to wake you up, throughout the day if you need a reboot, or at the end of the day if you want to get in an effective workout. For energy-boosting essential oils, the best methods of application are inhalation and topical applications of massage oils or creams. Inhaling essential oils can give you immediate, quick relief, whereas topical applications may take a little bit longer to affect you—but they will stay in your system for longer periods of time.

We will be using ginger, grapefruit, juniper, lemon, and peppermint for energy-boosting recipes. Some other common essential oils to boost energy are bergamot, eucalyptus, frankincense, geranium, lemongrass, lime, mandarin, orange, rosemary, and spearmint. If I need a quick pick-me-up, my favorites are peppermint, lemon, and orange. These essential oils are energy boosting, but they are not so stimulating that you can't focus.

## Essential Oils Can Help with Appetite

Eating is a necessity but overeating, snacking, and cravings are definitely not. When you are trying to manage your weight, you want to get a handle on these things. Essential oils can help decrease appetite and cravings. Overeating, snacking, and cravings can be caused by emotional imbalances, hormone imbalances, stress, mood swings, blood sugar imbalances, inflammation in the gut, and lack of sleep. This book includes essential oil recipes to help manage these urges. Remember, it is important that you eat throughout the day. The goal is not to starve yourself; the goal is to reduce between-meal cravings and the urge to overeat.

The first week of a diet can be exhausting mentally, physically, and emotionally, especially if you are reducing your calorie intake. Essential oils can help support you during these times. Intermittent fasting can

be effective for weight loss when done correctly. On intermittent fasting days, essential oils can help reduce cravings and appetite as well as give you extra energy. The most effective way to use essential oils for overeating, snacking, and cravings is to inhale the oil for five minutes before eating. You could inhale direct from the bottle, direct from the palms of your hands, or using a diffuser or inhaler. These blends are also effective when used topically, applied to the bottoms of your feet and your abdomen.

In this book, we will explore the uses of fennel, ginger, grapefruit, juniper, lavender, lemon, and peppermint. Some other essential oils that could help are basil, bergamot, cinnamon, lime, orange, patchouli, tea tree, and ylang-ylang. Cinnamon can be irritating to the skin, so please be cautious when using this essential oil topically.

## Essential Oils Can Spike Metabolism

Metabolism slows as you age, but it can also slow down if you are not consuming enough calories, not engaging in enough physical activity, not getting enough protein or vitamin D, not sleeping well, having hormone issues, or feeling stress. A slow metabolism can show up in a number of ways, including weight gain, headaches, cravings, digestive issues, depression, fatigue, food intolerances, dry skin, difficulty losing weight, and forgetfulness. While dieting, it is important to find natural ways to boost your metabolism. Along with essential oils, it is a good idea to work on deepening sleep, drinking more water, doing strength training, and making sure to eat the right amount of protein.

A sluggish metabolism and excess body fat can increase the risk and appearance of cellulite. Cellulite mainly occurs when your body has toxins it cannot get rid of. When trying to reduce the appearance of cellulite, it is important to use a massage oil with essential oils. Massaging the skin promotes drainage of the lymphatic system. The more you massage and increase circulation to the area, the more likely the cellulite will dissipate.

If you feel run-down, fatigued, like you have hit a plateau, or that you aren't losing any weight, essential oils could help you. They help increase circulation, stimulate your body, improve mood, promote detoxification, regulate digestion, and reduce cravings. Inhalation and topical applications are the best methods to spike metabolism. The oils can be inhaled using the bottle, the palms of your hands, a diffuser, or an inhaler. They can also be used topically, applied to the

bottoms of the feet, the abdomen, or massaged into the skin where cellulite is present.

The essential oils we will cover that improve metabolism are fennel, ginger, grapefruit, lemon, and peppermint. A few other options would be black pepper, cinnamon, and rosemary. Again, if you use cinnamon topically, please use caution.

▶ Make sure to see your physician for regular checkups. Seek medical attention immediately if you have any out-of-the-ordinary symptoms or believe you may be having a serious health issue. Safety always needs to come first. Essential oils can assist in symptom relief, but remember—they do not cure or treat any conditions.

## Essential Oils Can Alleviate Stress and Help You Sleep

Stress and sleep—where do I begin? When you are stressed, you don't sleep as well. And when you don't sleep as well, you become stressed. It is a vicious cycle.

If you are constantly stressed, your body is constantly in a fight-or-flight state. You only want your body to have a fight-or-flight response when you are in an emergency; "rest and digest" is where you want your body to be the majority of the time. When the body is resting and digesting, it can perform normal healing activities, including digesting the food you take in, eliminating what the body doesn't need, detoxing, breathing deeper, and slowing the heart rate.

Stress-reducing activities are not the same for everyone. One person might prefer yoga and meditation, whereas another person might prefer running and dancing. There are many stress-reducing activities you can try: candle gazing, walking, running, singing, dancing, spending time with friends and family, doing something that makes you laugh, sitting by a fire, deep breathing, artwork, positive affirmations, gratitude, progressive muscle relaxation, and—of course—using essential oils.

Improving sleep can be challenging, but it could change your life. We spend about one-third of our lives sleeping. When we sleep more deeply, our attitudes improve, we have more energy, we feel better, and our stress levels decrease. To improve your sleep, it is important to go to sleep and wake up at consistent times, decrease the amount of blue light exposure (especially before bed), reduce caffeine intake (especially in the evening), stop snacking before bed, meditate before bedtime, follow a nightly routine, and incorporate aromatherapy.

The essential oils we will cover that are best suited for stress relief are fennel, grapefruit, juniper, lavender, and lemon. The essential oils best suited for assisting sleep are grapefruit, juniper, lavender, and lemon. Some other very helpful options are basil, bergamot, cedarwood, clary sage, orange, patchouli, Roman chamomile, sandalwood, vetiver, and ylang-ylang. These can be used aromatically by inhalation or topical applications. A relaxing bath or shower with essential oils is a great way to unwind at the end of the day before going to bed. Other options would be using an inhaler, a diffuser, or applying essential oils to the bottoms of your feet, back of your neck, or as a massage oil.

## Essential Oils Can Help You Detox and Cleanse

Detoxing and cleansing means eliminating toxins that you take in with food and environment, or toxins that your body has accumulated over time.

Detoxing looks different from person to person, but in general terms, a detox is when you eliminate the main inflam-matory foods—including refined sugar, processed foods, gluten, trans and saturated fats, refined carbohydrates, alcohol, and dairy. Intermittent fasting, juice cleansing, fruit and vegetable detox, and clean food detox are a few examples of detox and cleanse pro-grams. When detoxing, make sure to focus on improving the quality of your sleep, discontinuing alcohol, improving stress response, adding in exercise, and drinking as much water as possible, as detoxing can dehydrate you. Detoxing activities might include dry brushing, oil pulling, drinking herbal teas, or sweating it out in a sauna.

Essential oils can significantly help your body's detoxification pro-cess. They can aid digestion so your body can eliminate properly, decrease inflammation so your body can absorb the necessary nutrients, and improve circulation and lymphatic drainage to decrease cellulite. The essential oils in this book that aid the body in detoxification are fennel, ginger, grapefruit, juniper, lavender, lemon, and peppermint. A few other helpful essential oils are frankincense, lemon-grass, oregano, patchouli, rosemary, and ylang-ylang. Topical applications are the most helpful. These essential oils can be used as a massage oil, body scrub, foot soak, bath salt, body wrap,

gel, cream, or even just diluted blends applied to the bottoms of the feet.

Keep in mind that essential oils can't do all of the work for you. They can aid you in the process, but they will not make the body detox and cleanse by itself.

Detox programs can be intimidating, stressful, and done incorrectly, so it is important to follow a program and be supervised by a physician or holistic provider. I once completed a detox in which I pushed myself too hard. I wasn't taking the cues my body was sending me, and I pushed through until the end. It caused me to have adrenal fatigue and worsened my acne. Most detoxes don't end that way, but they can if they are done incorrectly. As always, believ-ing in yourself will make this process so much easier. Go easy, trust the pro-cess, listen to your body, stay positive, and detox.

## Essential Oils Can Help You Find Balance

Balance can mean different things for different people. For me, having balance means being at peace, feeling happy, believing in myself, and being in tune with my mind, body, and soul. Balance has always been a goal of mine, and after 28 years, I finally feel like I have it and I am loving every minute!

To be unbalanced could mean feeling uneasy about where you are in life, striving for perfection, being too hard on yourself, feeling stressed, or not taking care of yourself.

It is essential to take time for self-care, find time to reset, and set realistic goals. Aromatherapy follows a holistic approach and wants us to consider the mind, body, and soul. Ask yourself some questions: Is my head in the right place? Are my goals realistic? Do I feel mentally healthy? Am I anxious? Do I feel stuck? Do I find time for myself? What goals do I have for my body? Have I hit a plateau? Do I feel physically healthy? Is my digestion regular? Do I trust the flow of life? Do I believe in

## LITTLE ADJUSTMENTS

Weight loss doesn't happen instantly; it takes time—so please be patient with yourself. You need to have a starting point, then gradually meet your goals and see the weight come off. Here are some steps and adjustments I highly recommend:

1. **Set realistic goals.** Reassess goals throughout your journey.

2. **Find some essential oil blends that can support you mentally and physically throughout your journey.**

3. **Start crowding out foods that no longer serve you.** Slowly replace processed foods with fresh fruits, fresh vegetables, smoothies, green juices, etc. Ideally, remove inflammatory foods so your body can absorb all of the nutrients you take in. Refined sugar, processed foods, gluten, trans and saturated fats, refined carbohydrates, alcohol, and dairy are the most inflammatory foods. It may not be realistic to remove all of those foods 100 percent of the time—the goal is to reduce your intake of these foods so you can look and feel healthy, improve digestion, boost your immune system, reduce muscle and joint pain, and so much more.

4. **Start slowly adding in exercise.** Exercise doesn't mean going to the gym and lifting weights or running on a treadmill every day. Exercise is any type of movement, and it is very important to make time for movement every day. Movement could mean yoga, walking, Pilates, weight lifting, swimming, running around the playground with your kids, dancing—really anything! Ideally, you will get at least 30 minutes of movement per day.

5. **Love your body.** No matter where you are in your journey, always believe in yourself because you can do anything you set your mind to. It takes being healthy on the inside and out to truly live a happy, healthy life.

myself? What am I grateful for? Do I give to others? Am I calm and peaceful?

These are some questions that can help you reflect to see how balanced your life is, as they bring in all three aspects: mind, body, and soul.

Essential oils we will cover in this book that relate to balance are fennel, ginger, grapefruit, juniper, lavender, lemon, and peppermint. Other essential oils that promote balance are bergamot, cedarwood, clary sage, frankincense, geranium, orange, patchouli, Roman chamomile, sandalwood, vetiver, and ylang-ylang. These essential oils can be used as inhalers, diffuser blends, bath salts, sprays, topically applied to the bottoms of the feet, wrists, or back of the neck, or used in neck and back massage.

## Blends in This Book

The blends in this book will be for increasing energy, suppressing appetite, boosting metabolism, relieving stress, promoting deep sleep, and encouraging detoxification and cleansing. We will go over a wide variety of applications, including bath salts, body oils, body wraps, creams, diffuser blends, inhalers, massage oils, roll-ons, shower steamers, and sprays.

Next, we will review seven essential oil profiles and learn the general benefits, precautions, and uses of each. I cannot wait to share how these essential oils can help you throughout your weight loss journey.

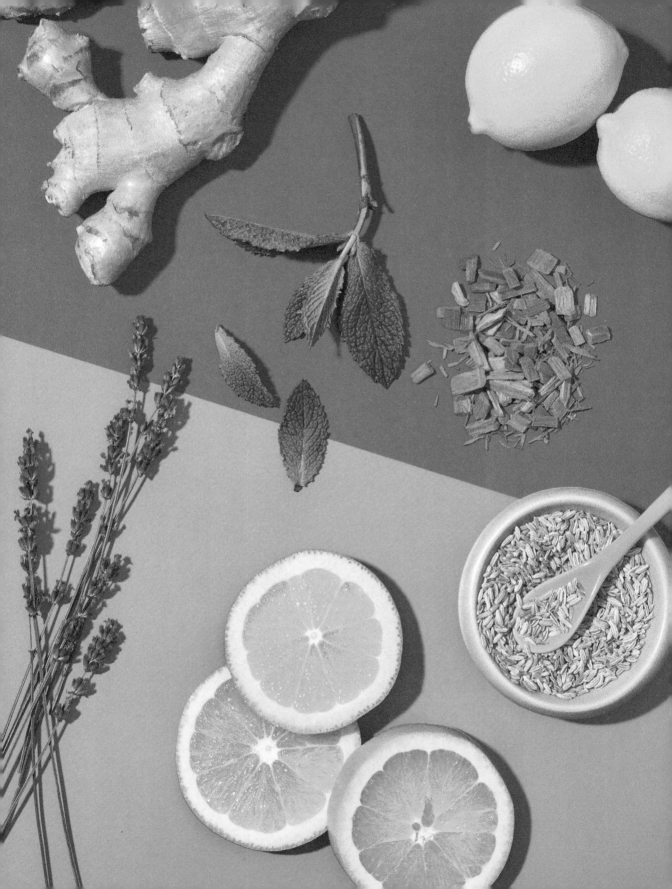

# profiles of essential oils for weight loss

This chapter includes profiles of most of the essential oils used in the blends in part 2. These profiles are important to review, as they include safety precautions, benefits, and recommended uses. Note that these essential oils are beneficial on their own as well as when combined in the recipes in part 2.

Remember, weight loss is not achieved solely by using these essential oils—but they *are* here to support you along the way by alleviating stress, curbing cravings, reducing the appearance of cellulite, increasing energy, kickstarting metabolism, regulating digestion, and relieving anxiety.

# fennel

*Foeniculum vulgare*

Seeds of the fennel plant are crushed and distilled to create the essential oil. Fennel is known for its digestive properties, relieving such conditions as indigestion, irritable bowel syndrome, excess gas, and constipation. Fennel is also beneficial for reducing inflammation and increasing energy.

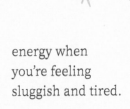

## PRECAUTIONS

Avoid use on children under five years of age, during pregnancy, while breastfeeding, and if you have an estrogen-dependent cancer or endometriosis. It can also cause skin sensitization if oxidized.

## BENEFITS

1. Aid metabolism
2. Alleviate bloating
3. Calm the overactive mind
4. Curb cravings
5. Decrease inflammation
6. Encourage healthy liver function
7. Improve circulation
8. Manage appetite
9. Promote mental focus
10. Reduce fluid retention
11. Regulate digestion

## BEST FOR

Appetite, calming, carminative, cellulite, detoxification, digestion, endocrine, focus, inflammation, metabolism, stress

## USES

Fennel essential oil promotes healthy digestion. If you are feeling bloated, constipated, or irregular, fennel is the oil for you. It can be applied directly to the skin, properly diluted, to aid metabolism, increase circulation, and regulate digestion. It can also be used aromatically to improve focus when concentration is lacking or boost energy when you're feeling sluggish and tired.

▶ Add to a diffuser or inhaler to curb cravings and decrease appetite.

▶ Add to a diffuser or inhaler to improve mental focus and concentration.

▶ Dilute with a carrier oil and massage onto areas where you are experiencing muscle or joint pain.

▶ Dilute with a carrier oil and massage onto your abdomen for digestive issues. Massage in a clockwise direction for constipation and counterclockwise for diarrhea.

# ginger

*Zingiber officinale*

Ginger essential oil is distilled from the root of the plant. It is best known for reducing inflammation in the gut so your body can absorb nutrients you are taking in. It also has many benefits for energy, focus, and mental health. Since it has a warming effect and is distilled from the root of the plant, it offers support and strength to get through difficult times.

## PRECAUTIONS

No known
safety concerns

## BENEFITS

1. Aid digestion
2. Boost metabolism
3. Clear the mind
4. Curb cravings
5. Encourage focus
6. Energize
7. Flush toxins
8. Increase motivation
9. Promote grounding
10. Reduce inflammation
11. Relieve nausea

## BEST FOR

Appetite, carminative, clarity, detoxification, digestion, energy, focus, inflammation, metabolism, motivation, nausea, pain

## USES

Ginger essential oil can be used to aid digestion and boost metabolism when massaged onto the abdomen. When used aromatically, you will feel stronger, more grounded, and have more mental clarity and focus. It is also helpful for controlling cravings that arise in your weight loss journey. I love using ginger during times of transition, when I need clarity, support, or grounding.

▸ Add to a bath to kickstart your metabolism.

▸ Add to a diffuser or inhaler to curb cravings.

▸ During times of change, add ginger essential oil to a diffuser to get the clarity that you need.

▸ Massage onto the abdomen with a carrier oil to improve digestion. Massage in a clockwise direction for constipation and counterclockwise for diarrhea.

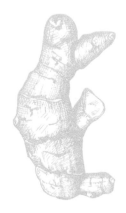

# grapefruit

*Citrus × paradisi*

Grapefruit is expressed or distilled from the peel of the fruit. It is well known for its uplifting properties to energize and reduce symptoms of anxiety and depression. Grapefruit essential oil aids digestion and boosts your body's metabolism.

## PRECAUTIONS

Expressed grapefruit essential oil is photo-toxic, meaning you should avoid direct sunlight and tanning beds for 12 hours after using it. Skin reactions can occur if the oil is oxidized, so make sure to store the oil in a cool, dark place, preferably the refrigerator.

## BENEFITS

1. Alleviate stress
2. Boost mood during hard times
3. Break down fat
4. Increase energy
5. Kickstart metabolism
6. Manage appetite and cravings
7. Promote lymphatic drainage
8. Reduce cellulite
9. Reduce fluid retention
10. Regulate digestion
11. Relieve anxiety and depression symptoms

## BEST FOR

Anxiety, appetite, calming, cellulite, depression, detoxification, digestion, energy, metabolism, sleep, stress

## USES

Grapefruit essential oil can be used right away in the morning to boost energy and work as a natural appetite suppressant for the whole day. It can be massaged onto the skin to reduce the appearance of cellulite and fat in the body. Grapefruit also balances the mood—if you feel anxious or depressed, go get your bottle of grapefruit essential oil.

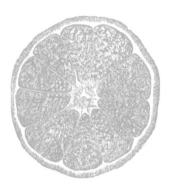

▸ Add to a bath to alleviate stress and unwind from the day.

▸ Add to a diffuser or inhaler to boost energy levels.

▸ Dilute with a carrier oil and massage onto areas with cellulite.

▸ Use in a diffuser or inhaler to control your appetite and curb cravings.

# juniper berry

*Juniperus communis*

Juniper berry essential oil is distilled from the berries of the tree. It is known for detoxifying and cleansing the body. It is also great for cleansing and clearing the air and the skin. When digestion concerns arise—such as constipation, diarrhea, cramping, and excess gas—juniper berry essential oil can help.

## PRECAUTIONS

Skin sensitization can occur if the oil has oxidized, so it is important to keep this oil in a cool, dark place, preferably the refrigerator.

## BENEFITS

1. Boost energy
2. Calm the nervous system
3. Control appetite
4. Curb cravings
5. Decrease bloating
6. Eliminate toxins
7. Reduce cellulite
8. Reduce fluid retention
9. Regulate digestion
10. Relieve anxiety and stress
11. Support liver and kidney function

## BEST FOR

Anxiety, appetite, bloating, calming, cellulite, detoxification, digestion, energy, fluid retention, inflammation, pain, relaxation, sleep, stress

## USES

Topically, juniper berry essential oil is great for promoting detoxification and eliminating toxins from your body. When used aromatically, it helps calm and ground you while controlling appetite and curbing cravings. Throughout your weight loss journey, it is important to stay balanced, and juniper berry can help you with that.

▶ Add to a diffuser or inhaler to control cravings.

▶ Diffuse during times of stress or during meditation to deepen your connection.

▶ Dilute and massage onto areas where cellulite is present.

▶ Dilute and use as a massage oil to clear the skin of impurities and calm the nervous system.

# lavender

*Lavandula angustifolia* or *Lavandula officinalis*

Lavender essential oil is distilled from the flowering tops of the plant. Lavender is a popular oil due to its versatility. It is very mild and promotes relaxation as soon as the bottle is opened. Weight loss journeys can bring up stress, fear, and anxiety, which can greatly affect sleep. If you aren't sleeping well, it is hard to lose weight. Lavender is a great oil for improving sleep.

## PRECAUTIONS

No known
safety concerns.

## BENEFITS

1. Alleviate headaches
2. Calm the nervous stomach
3. Control overeating
4. Curb cravings
5. Ease anxiety and depression
6. Improve cellulite
7. Promote deep sleep
8. Quiet the overactive mind
9. Reduce inflammation
10. Regulate digestion
11. Relieve muscle and joint pain

## BEST FOR

Anxiety, appetite, calming, cellulite, depression, detoxification, digestion, inflammation, relaxation, sleep, stress

## USES

Lavender essential oil is good for almost anything! Its main use with regard to promoting weight loss is easing the mind. This oil is here to be your sidekick throughout your journey. It can be applied topically to regulate digestion, ease the mind, reduce inflammation, promote deep sleep, and alleviate headaches. It can be used aromatically for controlling cravings and overeating, calming the mind, and easing anxiety and depression.

▸ **Add to a bath to promote deep sleep and relaxation.**

▸ **Add to a diffuser or inhaler to reduce stress and anxiety that arise throughout the day.**

▸ **Apply diluted to your abdomen to calm your nervous stomach.**

▸ **Create a diluted massage oil to relieve muscle and joint pain.**

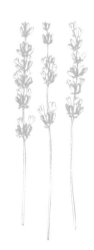

# lemon

*Citrus × limon*

Lemon peels are expressed or distilled to create lemon essential oil. The scent is refreshing and uplifting, calming the overactive mind. It is a versatile oil and can be used for mental, emotional, and physical concerns. It naturally detoxifies the body and reduces fluid retention.

## PRECAUTIONS

Expressed lemon essential oil is phototoxic, meaning you should avoid direct sunlight and tanning beds for 12 hours after using it. Skin reactions can occur if the oil is oxidized, so make sure to store the oil in a cool, dark place, preferably the refrigerator.

## BENEFITS

1. Alleviate stress
2. Boost energy
3. Control appetite
4. Curb cravings
5. Decrease inflammation
6. Ease anxiety and depression
7. Eliminate toxins
8. Reduce cellulite
9. Reduce fluid retention
10. Spike metabolism
11. Uplift your spirits

## BEST FOR

Anxiety, appetite, calming, cellulite, depression, detoxification, digestion, energy, fluid retention, focus, inflammation, metabolism, motivation, sleep, stress

## USES

Try to go easy on yourself throughout your journey. If you are struggling to be positive, inhale lemon essential oil using a diffuser or inhaler. It can increase motivation, improve focus, boost energy, and calm fears. Inhaling lemon essential oil can also curb cravings and control overeating.

▶ Add to a bath to unwind and clear the mind.

▶ Add to a diffuser or inhaler for an energy boost pre-workout.

▶ Dilute with a carrier oil and massage onto areas where cellulite is present.

▶ Massage onto the abdomen with a carrier oil to reduce fluid retention and promote healthy digestion.

# peppermint

*Mentha × piperita*

Peppermint essential oil is distilled from the leaves of the plant. It is an energizing oil, but not so energizing that you lose focus. It is mostly known for its digestive and anti-inflammatory properties. Regulating digestion is important throughout your weight loss journey—you need to be able to eliminate the food you are taking in as well as any toxins your body has stored over time.

### PRECAUTIONS

Do not apply on or near the face of infants or children. Avoid use on children under five years of age.

### BENEFITS

1. Boost energy
2. Calm muscle spasms
3. Cleanse the lymphatic system
4. Clear the mind
5. Decrease inflammation
6. Eliminate toxins
7. Improve focus
8. Motivate you to move your body
9. Regulate digestion
10. Soothe an upset stomach
11. Suppress cravings

### BEST FOR

Appetite, carminative, detoxification, digestion, energy, focus, inflammation, metabolism, motivation, pain

### USES

Peppermint essential oil can be applied, properly diluted, directly to the abdomen to promote regular digestion as well as soothe an upset or nervous stomach. It can be used aromatically to curb cravings and control appetite. Peppermint is my go-to for pre-workout—it gives me the drive and motivation I need when I am feeling sluggish.

▸ Add to a diffuser or inhaler before your workout to feel energized, focused, and motivated.

▸ Add to a diffuser or inhaler to control appetite and fight cravings.

▸ Add to an unscented lotion and massage onto areas where you are experiencing muscle or joint pain.

▸ Massage onto the abdomen to regulate digestion or soothe an upset stomach. Massage in a clockwise direction for constipation and counterclockwise for diarrhea.

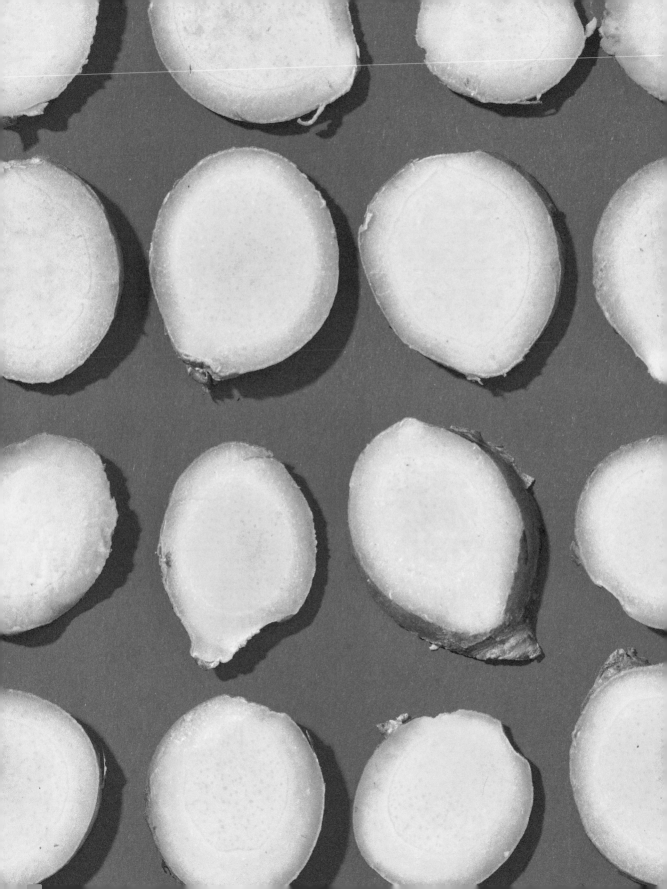

# part II

# BLENDS FOR BOOSTING WEIGHT LOSS

Now that we've established a foundation for working with essential oils—learning about how to store and use them safely as well as which ones can specifically aid your weight loss process—it's time to learn about blends.

In this part of the book, you'll find a wide variety of blends, including recipes for inhalers, diffusers, massage oils, rollers, creams, gels, scrubs, spritzers, body washes, bath salts, and more—all designed to support you as you work on losing weight. There are blends to naturally manage appetite, spike metabolism, boost energy, encourage detoxification, improve digestion, enhance deep sleep, and promote calm.

You can benefit from these blends even after you reach your weight loss goals. Stay motivated, believe in yourself, be patient, and keep pushing.

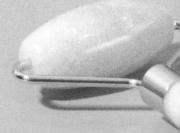

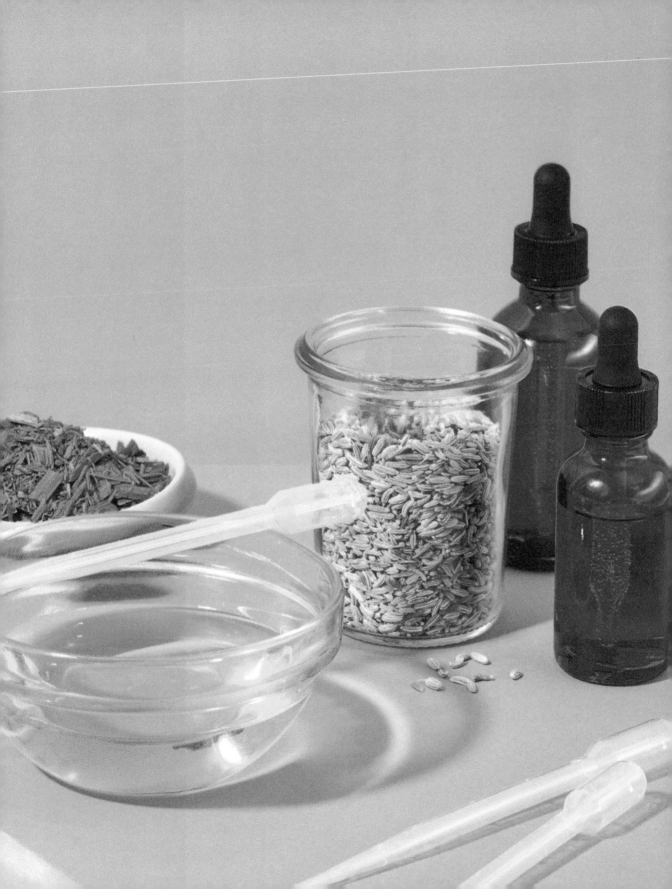

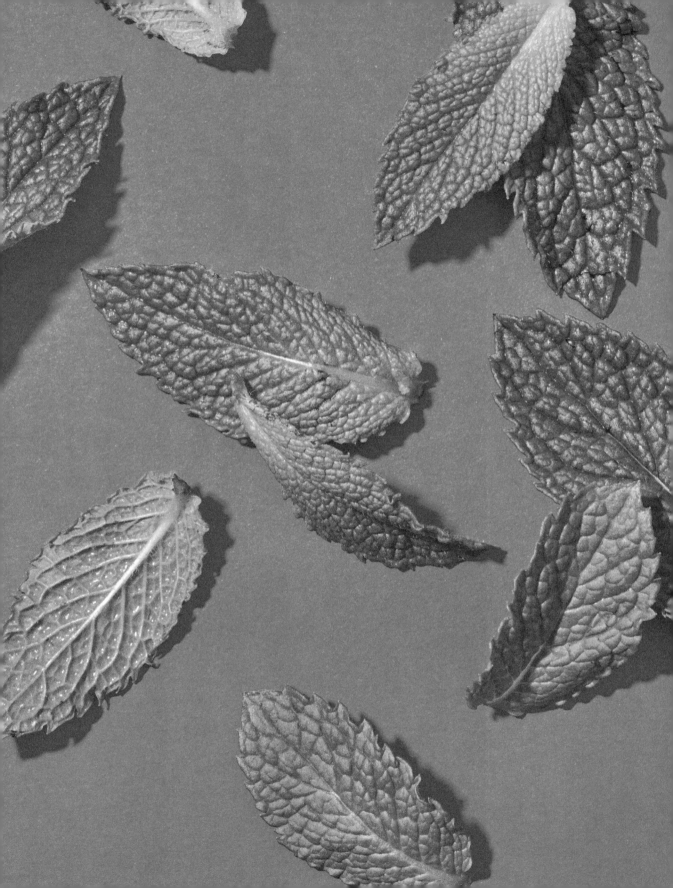

# 4

# appetite & metabolism

# appetite management diffuser blend

When you are feeling hungry despite having just eaten, this diffuser blend is a great choice. It's also helpful during intermittent fasting days when you are fighting hunger or if you are reducing your calorie intake. It is a great way to curb hunger, increase productivity, and boost energy levels. I love diffusing this blend first thing in the morning to boost energy levels and reduce unnecessary hunger throughout the day.

1 (10-milliliter) euro dropper bottle

2 plastic pipettes

125 drops grapefruit oil

85 drops lemon oil

Diffuser

▸ Makes: 10 milliliters (approximately 20 uses)

▸ Indirect inhalation

▸ Safe for all ages

1. Using the plastic pipettes, add the essential oils to the 10-milliliter euro dropper bottle.

2. Reinsert the orifice reducer that came with the bottle, secure the cap, and gently swirl the bottle for about 1 minute. Label the bottle.

3. Add 8 to 12 drops to your diffuser and diffuse in 30-minute increments.

4. Enjoy and resist the urge!

# give yourself grace diffuser blend

It is hard to resist cravings and hunger, and you need to be gentle with yourself. Don't let your thoughts race or make you feel like a failure. Instead, put this blend in your diffuser, relax, let your mind clear, and continue on with your day. The essential oils in this blend will help decrease hunger for your next meal. I didn't create this blend so we can overeat every meal and forget about it—I created this blend for the occasional meal we struggle to stop eating.

1 (10-milliliter) euro dropper bottle

3 plastic pipettes

50 drops ginger oil

65 drops lavender oil

95 drops lemon oil

Diffuser

▸ Makes: 10 milliliters (approximately 20 uses)

▸ Indirect inhalation

▸ Safe for all ages

1. Using the plastic pipettes, add the essential oils to the 10-milliliter euro dropper bottle.

2. Reinsert the orifice reducer that came with the bottle, secure the cap, and gently swirl the bottle for about 1 minute. Label the bottle.

3. Add 8 to 12 drops to your diffuser and diffuse in 30-minute increments.

4. Enjoy and give yourself grace!

# kick cravings diffuser blend

Cravings can be caused by a number of things, including lack of nutrients, addiction (yes, sugar is extremely addicting!), imbalanced hormones, and strong emotions. This diffuser blend is multipurpose, as both peppermint and fennel work to fight cravings as well as energize, promote focus, regulate digestion, and clear the sinuses. In general, I do not consume artificial sugar, but when I do, I crave artificial sugar like crazy for at least two weeks. I love using this blend when those cravings arise.

1 (10-milliliter) euro dropper bottle

2 plastic pipettes

130 drops fennel oil

80 drops peppermint oil

Diffuser

▸ Makes: 10 milliliters (approximately 20 uses)

▸ Indirect inhalation

▸ Safe for ages 5+

⚠ Avoid use during pregnancy, while breastfeeding, and if you have an estrogen-dependent cancer or endometriosis.

1. Using the plastic pipettes, add the essential oils to the 10-milliliter euro dropper bottle.

2. Reinsert the orifice reducer that came with the bottle, secure the cap, and gently swirl the bottle for about 1 minute. Label the bottle.

3. Add 8 to 12 drops to your diffuser and diffuse in 30-minute increments.

4. Enjoy and kick those cravings!

# kickstart your metabolism diffuser blend

Metabolism is the way your body processes food and converts it into energy. This blend will help kickstart or speed up your metabolism so you can burn more calories and shed unwanted weight. I love to use this blend right after I eat to help process the food and increase my energy level and focus.

1 (10-milliliter) euro dropper bottle

3 plastic pipettes

50 drops fennel oil

90 drops grapefruit oil

70 drops lemon oil

Diffuser

▸ Makes: 10 milliliters (approximately 20 uses)

▸ Indirect inhalation

▸ Safe for ages 5+

⚠ Avoid use during pregnancy, while breastfeeding, or if you have an estrogen-dependent cancer or endometriosis.

1. Using the plastic pipettes, add the essential oils to the 10-milliliter euro dropper bottle.

2. Reinsert the orifice reducer that came with the bottle, secure the cap, and gently swirl the bottle for about 1 minute. Label the bottle.

3. Add 8 to 12 drops to your diffuser and diffuse in 30-minute increments.

4. Enjoy and kickstart your metabolism!

# stop overeating diffuser blend

Do you find yourself overeating at meals? Or do you find yourself eating because you are bored? This blend works best when diffused at least 10 minutes before you sit down to eat. When trying to lose weight, it is important to eat mindfully. Sit down, focus on what you are eating, think about all of the nutrients you are taking in, chew each bite at least 30 times, and eat slowly.

1 (10-milliliter) euro dropper bottle

3 plastic pipettes

40 drops grapefruit oil

60 drops lavender oil

110 drops lemon oil

Diffuser

▸ Makes: 10 milliliters (approximately 20 uses)

▸ Indirect inhalation

▸ Safe for all ages

1. Using the plastic pipettes, add the essential oils to the 10-milliliter euro dropper bottle.

2. Reinsert the orifice reducer that came with the bottle, secure the cap, and gently swirl the bottle for about 1 minute. Label the bottle.

3. Add 8 to 12 drops to your diffuser and diffuse in 30-minute increments.

4. Enjoy and eat mindfully!

# curb sugar cravings inhaler

Sugar is extremely addicting, and once you give your body sugar, all it wants is more. When you are making diet changes, sugar cravings can be stronger than normal because your body wants what it knows. When cravings hit, think before you snack—consider what sugar does to your body and go get your inhaler. Sugar causes weight gain and fatigue, and can negatively affect your blood sugar, teeth, skin, liver, kidneys, stomach, joints, pancreas, and even your heart.

**Blank inhaler**

**3 plastic pipettes**

**12 drops grapefruit oil**

**13 drops juniper oil**

**5 drops peppermint oil**

▸ Makes: 1 inhaler

▸ Direct inhalation

▸ Safe for ages 5+

1. Using the plastic pipettes, mix the essential oils in a small glass bowl.

2. Remove the cover on the inhaler tube. Using tweezers, place the wick in the bowl of essential oils and move it around until the essential oils are absorbed.

3. Use tweezers to place the moistened wick back in the inhaler tube.

4. Put the cover back on to secure the wick. Label the inhaler.

5. Twist off the cap and inhale the aroma for 2 to 5 minutes at a time.

6. Enjoy and curb those cravings!

# increase appetite inhaler

During your weight loss journey, it is important to eat throughout the day. You may think skipping meals is an easy way to lose weight, but your body needs fuel. When you skip meals, your metabolism and digestion can slow. At your next meal, your body is sluggish and struggles to process food, absorb nutrients, and eliminate toxins. If you aren't hungry and it has been a while since your last meal, use this inhaler and go find a healthy snack, such as fresh fruit or vegetables. This will provide your body with incredible nutrients and keep your metabolism and digestion moving.

**Blank inhaler**

**2 plastic pipettes**

**18 drops ginger oil**

**12 drops peppermint oil**

▸ Makes: 1 inhaler

▸ Direct inhalation

▸ Safe for ages 5+

1. Using the plastic pipettes, mix the essential oils in a small glass bowl.

2. Remove the cover on the inhaler tube. Using tweezers, place the wick in the bowl of essential oils and move it around until the essential oils are absorbed.

3. Use tweezers to place the moistened wick back in the inhaler tube.

4. Put the cover back on to secure the wick. Label the inhaler.

5. Twist off the cap and inhale the aroma for 2 to 5 minutes at a time.

6. Enjoy a healthy snack!

# pre-meal inhaler

Are you eating a meal that isn't super nutritious? This pre-meal inhaler promotes healthy digestion and reduces the risk of indigestion, upset stomach, diarrhea, and excess gas. It is impossible to eat clean and nutritious food 100 percent of the time—no one can. Don't obsess over it. When you have a meal that isn't necessarily serving your body, eat slowly and mindfully, and be sure you've got this inhaler! It will help reduce the possible side effects so you can go about your day as usual.

**Blank inhaler**

**3 plastic pipettes**

**9 drops fennel oil**

**14 drops ginger oil**

**7 drops juniper oil**

▸ Makes: 1 inhaler

▸ Direct inhalation

▸ Safe for ages 5+

⚠ Avoid use during pregnancy, while breastfeeding, and if you have an estrogen-dependent cancer or endometriosis.

1. Using the plastic pipettes, mix the essential oils in a small glass bowl.

2. Remove the cover on the inhaler tube. Using tweezers, place the wick in the bowl of essential oils and move it around until the essential oils are absorbed.

3. Use tweezers to place the moistened wick back in the inhaler tube.

4. Put the cover back on to secure the wick. Label the inhaler.

5. Twist off the cap and inhale the aroma for 2 to 5 minutes at a time.

6. Enjoy and eat clean when possible!

# stop mindless snacking inhaler

Eating mindlessly can sabotage your weight loss journey. I do not recommend eating in front of a computer or phone—being distracted makes it easy to overeat or eat too quickly. Also, when you are bored or tired, don't eat! Find something else to do, like going for a walk, dancing, taking a shower, doing meal prep, grocery shopping—anything but eating. Eating when you are bored is an easy way to snack too often. This inhaler can help you decrease snacking when it isn't necessary. And always remember to eat mindfully.

**Blank inhaler**

**3 plastic pipettes**

**9 drops juniper oil**

**15 drops lemon oil**

**6 drops peppermint oil**

▶ Makes: 1 inhaler

▶ Direct Inhalation

▶ Safe for ages 5+

1. Using the plastic pipettes, mix the essential oils in a small glass bowl.

2. Remove the cover on the inhaler tube. Using tweezers, place the wick in the bowl of essential oils and move it around until the essential oils are absorbed.

3. Use tweezers to place the moistened wick back in the inhaler tube.

4. Put the cover back on to secure the wick. Label the inhaler.

5. Twist off the cap and inhale the aroma for 2 to 5 minutes at a time.

6. Enjoy and stop mindless snacking!

# metabolism boost massage oil

This blend can be used at any time during the day. To boost your metabolism most efficiently, it is best to start the day with a shower, alternating hot and cold water, followed by this massage oil. The essential oils in this blend are energizing and, when used topically, they penetrate the skin and get into the bloodstream so the molecules can disperse throughout the body.

**1 (2-ounce) glass dropper bottle**

**3 plastic pipettes**

**22 drops ginger oil**

**26 drops grapefruit oil**

**24 drops lemon oil**

**2 ounces carrier oil of your choice**

▸ Makes: 2 ounces

▸ Topical use

▸ Safe for ages 5+

⚠ Do not use for 12 hours before being in direct sunlight or a tanning bed.

1. Using the plastic pipettes, add the essential oils to the 2-ounce glass dropper bottle.

2. Twist the cap on and gently swirl the bottle for about 1 minute.

3. Add the carrier oil, cover, and gently swirl the bottle for about 2 minutes to blend. Label the bottle.

4. Massage onto the abdomen in a clockwise motion. If you can reach or have someone else massage the oil blend onto your back, that is also beneficial.

5. Enjoy and boost your metabolism!

# craving crusher roller

Cravings can come at inconvenient times. Keep this roller in your purse or pocket so you can bring it everywhere you go. When cravings hit, you will know what to do. A craving is difficult to crush, so be gentle with yourself, confident that you can kick it, and mindful if you choose to eat.

1 (10-milliliter) roll-on bottle

4 plastic pipettes

2 drops fennel oil

4 drops juniper oil

2 drops lavender oil

10 milliliters carrier oil of your choice

▸ Makes: 10 milliliters

▸ Topical use

▸ Safe for ages 5+

⚠ Avoid use during pregnancy, while breastfeeding, and if you have an estrogen-dependent cancer or endometriosis.

1. Using the plastic pipettes, add the essential oils to the 10-milliliter roll-on bottle. Twist the cap on and gently swirl the bottle for about 1 minute.

2. Add the carrier oil, cover, and gently swirl the bottle for about 2 minutes to blend. Label the bottle.

3. Roll onto the bottoms of your feet, onto your abdomen in a clockwise motion, and onto your wrists so you can inhale anytime you need.

4. Enjoy and crush those cravings!

# metabolism lift roller

This roller is convenient for on-the-go or at-home use. I love to use this blend every morning so my metabolism starts off with a bang. It is easy to apply and very effective at increasing metabolism, regulating digestion, energizing, and grounding.

1 (10-milliliter)
roll-on bottle

4 plastic pipettes

2 drops ginger oil

5 drops grapefruit oil

1 drop juniper oil

10 milliliters carrier oil
of your choice

▸ Makes: 10 milliliters

▸ Topical use

▸ Safe for ages 5+

⚠ Do not use for
12 hours before being
in direct sunlight or
a tanning bed.

1. Using the plastic pipettes, add the essential oils to the 10-milliliter roll-on bottle. Twist the cap on and gently swirl the bottle for about 1 minute.

2. Add the carrier oil, cover, and gently swirl the bottle for about 2 minutes to blend. Label the bottle.

3. Roll onto the bottoms of your feet, onto your abdomen in a clockwise motion, and onto your wrists so you can inhale anytime you need.

4. Enjoy and lift your metabolism!

# overeating control roller

It's not hard to overeat. Do you eat in front of the TV, computer, or phone? Do you eat while working? Do you pay attention to what you are eating? This essential oil blend can help control your appetite when used in combination with slow, mindful eating. Do you want even more benefits? Eat fresh fruits and vegetables whenever possible—especially before eating a full meal.

1 (10-milliliter) roll-on bottle

4 plastic pipettes

4 drops fennel oil

3 drops lavender oil

1 drop peppermint oil

10 milliliters carrier oil of your choice

▸ Makes: 10 milliliters

▸ Topical use

▸ Safe for ages 5+

⚠ Avoid use during pregnancy, while breastfeeding, and if you have an estrogen-dependent cancer or endometriosis.

1. Using the plastic pipettes, add the essential oils to the 10-milliliter roll-on bottle. Twist the cap on and gently swirl the bottle for about 1 minute.

2. Add the carrier oil, cover, and gently swirl the bottle for about 2 minutes to blend. Label the bottle.

3. Roll onto the bottoms of your feet, onto your abdomen in a clockwise motion, and onto your wrists so you can inhale anytime you need. Apply at least 10 minutes prior to eating.

4. Enjoy and resist overeating!

# resist the urge roller

This versatile roller can be used for multiple urges such as overeating, cravings, snacking, and mindless eating. Whatever your urge is, this blend can help! It also boosts energy levels and promotes calm thoughts. When using this blend, try saying a positive affirmation. When I get a sugar craving, for instance, I use this blend and say things like, "I am satisfied. I have power over this craving. I love my body."

1 (10-milliliter) roll-on bottle

4 plastic pipettes

4 drops grapefruit oil

3 drops juniper oil

1 drop lavender oil

10 milliliters carrier oil of your choice

▸ Makes: 10 milliliters

▸ Topical use

▸ Safe for ages 5+

⚠ Do not use for 12 hours before being in direct sunlight or a tanning bed.

1. Using the plastic pipettes, add the essential oils to the 10-milliliter roll-on bottle. Twist the cap on and gently swirl the bottle for about 1 minute.

2. Add the carrier oil, cover, and gently swirl the bottle for about 2 minutes to blend. Label the bottle.

3. Roll onto the bottoms of your feet, onto your abdomen in a clockwise motion, and onto your wrists so you can inhale anytime you need. Apply at least 10 minutes prior to eating.

4. Enjoy and resist the urge!

# stop snacking hand cream

If I have lotion on my hands, I don't eat unless I get up and wash my hands first. If this sounds like you, give this recipe a try! Not only does this hand cream make you think twice about snacking, but it also contains essential oils that help curb cravings. Snacking is easy to do and can negate the work you're doing to lose weight. Always have fresh fruits, vegetables, and healthy snacks prepared and ready to eat. And if you just ate but you still want a snack, use this hand cream.

1 (2-ounce) plastic squeeze bottle with flip top

3 plastic pipettes

11 drops ginger oil

16 drops lavender oil

5 drops peppermint oil

2 ounces unscented lotion

▸ Makes: 2 ounces

▸ Topical use

▸ Safe for ages 5+

1. Using the plastic pipettes, add the essential oils to a small glass bowl and stir to mix them together.

2. Add the unscented lotion to the bowl and stir until combined. This may take a couple of minutes.

3. Use a spoon to pour the lotion and oil mixture into the 2-ounce squeeze bottle. Label the bottle.

4. Rub onto hands when you feel like snacking.

5. Enjoy and don't give in!

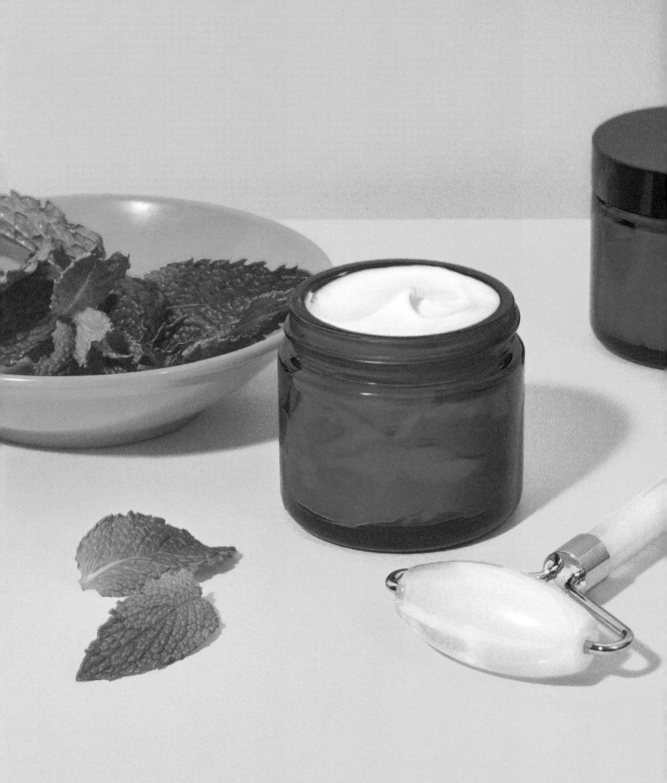

# energy

# boosting diffuser blend

When your diet and exercise routine change, your body can feel more fatigued than usual. You might have resorted to using caffeine in the past. While caffeine is great for an immediate boost, you'll crash later. With essential oils, you don't experience the crash. This blend has an amazing aroma and gives you the boost you need to continue with your day. When your energy is increased, you are more productive and can find energy without caffeine.

1 (10-milliliter) euro dropper bottle

2 plastic pipettes

120 drops juniper oil

90 drops peppermint oil

Diffuser

▸ Makes: 10 milliliters (approximately 20 uses)

▸ Indirect inhalation

▸ Safe for ages 5+

1. Using the plastic pipettes, add the essential oils to the 10-milliliter euro dropper bottle.

2. Reinsert the orifice reducer that came with the bottle, secure the cap, and gently swirl the bottle for about 1 minute. Label the bottle.

3. Add 8 to 12 drops to your diffuser and diffuse in 30-minute increments.

4. Enjoy and feel energized!

# citrus energy diffuser blend

Citrus essential oils are known for their energizing, balancing, mood-boosting, immune-enhancing, cleansing, and respiratory-clearing properties. These essential oils can be used throughout the day—they are safe for everyone and positively affect anyone in the room where the diffuser is. Plus, when diffused, these oils are also cleaning and freshening the air, sanitizing surfaces, boosting immune systems, and easing anxiety.

1 (10-milliliter) euro dropper bottle

2 plastic pipettes

105 drops grapefruit oil

105 drops lemon oil

Diffuser

▸ Makes: 10 milliliters (approximately 20 uses)

▸ Indirect inhalation

▸ Safe for all ages

1. Using the plastic pipettes, add the essential oils to the 10-milliliter euro dropper bottle.

2. Reinsert the orifice reducer that came with the bottle, secure the cap, and gently swirl the bottle for about 1 minute. Label the bottle.

3. Add 8 to 12 drops to your diffuser and diffuse in 30-minute increments.

4. Enjoy and get on your feet!

# second wind diffuser blend

Do you start your day off energized, then feel fatigued by mid-morning or mid-afternoon? This could be caused by poor-quality sleep, not enough sleep, overeating, seasonal changes, or diet and exercise changes. This diffuser blend is here for you during those times of fatigue. Avoid taking naps, because that can negatively affect your quality of sleep at night. Instead, turn on your diffuser, feel energized, and be productive.

1 (10-milliliter) euro dropper bottle

3 plastic pipettes

65 drops grapefruit oil

105 drops lemon oil

40 drops peppermint oil

Diffuser

▶ Makes: 10 milliliters (approximately 20 uses)

▶ Indirect inhalation

▶ Safe for ages 5+

1. Using the plastic pipettes, add the essential oils to the 10-milliliter euro dropper bottle.

2. Reinsert the orifice reducer that came with the bottle, secure the cap, and gently swirl the bottle for about 1 minute. Label the bottle.

3. Add 8 to 12 drops to your diffuser and diffuse in 30-minute increments.

4. Enjoy and get a second wind!

# pre-workout salt inhaler

This salt inhaler is perfect for just before you exercise and can also be used for an energy boost or to clear your respiratory system when you are congested or sick. Before your workouts, take 2 to 5 minutes for deep breathing. Focus on your chest and stomach expanding and contracting while inhaling the aroma from this inhaler. Not only does this kind of deep breathing improve breath control for a more effective workout, but the essential oils in this blend (plus the salt in the inhaler) help open the lungs for even greater breath control throughout your exercise routine.

1 (10-milliliter) euro dropper bottle

3 plastic pipettes

9 drops fennel oil

12 drops lemon oil

9 drops peppermint oil

Himalayan salt (texture can be coarse or fine)

▸ Makes: 10 milliliters

▸ Direct inhalation

▸ Safe for ages 5+

⚠ Avoid use during pregnancy, while breastfeeding, and if you have an estrogen-dependent cancer or endometriosis.

1. Using the plastic pipettes, add the essential oils to the 10-milliliter bottle. Twist the cap on and swirl the bottle for about 1 minute to blend.

2. Remove the cap and add the Himalayan salt.

3. Discard the orifice reducer, twist the cap on tightly and shake for about 2 minutes. Label the bottle.

4. Remove the cap and waft under your nose while taking deep breaths for 2 to 5 minutes. Use up to 4 times daily.

5. Enjoy and get moving!

# wake me up inhaler

I used to be envious of morning people, and then I created this inhaler. It sits on my nightstand, and I use it the second my alarm goes off to perk me up more quickly when I wake up. This is also useful throughout the day when you are feeling sluggish and fatigued. I like to incorporate positive affirmations when I use this inhaler. As you breathe in the scent, say things like, "I am a morning person. I am energized. I am ready to take on the day. I feel refreshed."

**Blank inhaler**

**3 plastic pipettes**

**10 drops juniper oil**

**13 drops lemon oil**

**7 drops peppermint oil**

▸ Makes: 1 inhaler

▸ Direct inhalation

▸ Safe for ages 5+

1. Using the plastic pipettes, mix the essential oils in a small glass bowl.

2. Remove the cover on the inhaler tube. Using tweezers, place the wick in the bowl of essential oils and move it around until the essential oils are absorbed.

3. Use tweezers to place the moistened wick back in the inhaler tube.

4. Put the cover back on to secure the wick. Label the inhaler.

5. Twist off the cap and inhale the aroma for 2 to 5 minutes at a time.

6. Enjoy and wake up!

# post-workout massage oil

Do you exercise regularly or are you trying to exercise more? That's great! Exercise can cause soreness, muscle pain, joint pain, fatigue, tightness, and tense muscles. This massage oil helps your muscles recover from your workout naturally so you can continue your day and be ready for an effective workout tomorrow. Ginger can cause a slight warming sensation and peppermint a cooling sensation, so if you feel either when using this massage oil, that is completely normal.

1 (2-ounce) glass dropper bottle

3 plastic pipettes

24 drops ginger oil

30 drops lavender oil

18 drops peppermint oil

2 ounces carrier oil of your choice

▸ Makes: 2 ounces

▸ Topical use

▸ Safe for ages 5+

1. Using the plastic pipettes, add the essential oils to the 2-ounce glass dropper bottle.

2. Twist the cap on and gently swirl the bottle for about 1 minute.

3. Add the carrier oil, cover, and gently swirl the bottle for about 2 minutes to blend. Label the bottle.

4. Rub and massage this blend into sore and tight muscles. If you can reach or have someone else massage the oil blend onto your back, that is also beneficial.

5. Enjoy and recover!

# vital energy body oil

Body oils penetrate deeper into the skin when used after a warm shower or bath, because your pores are open and ready to receive nutrients. This helps deliver the essential oil molecules into the bloodstream, providing you with energy. Body oils also act as a barrier to keep your skin smooth and hydrated.

1 (2-ounce) glass dropper bottle

3 plastic pipettes

16 drops grapefruit oil

14 drops juniper oil

18 drops lemon oil

2 ounces carrier oil of your choice

▸ Makes: 2 ounces

▸ Topical use

▸ Safe for ages 5+

⚠ Do not use for 12 hours before being in direct sunlight or a tanning bed.

1. Using the plastic pipettes, add the essential oils to the 2-ounce glass dropper bottle.

2. Twist the cap on and swirl gently for about 1 minute.

3. Add the carrier oil, cover, and gently swirl the bottle for about 2 minutes to blend. Label the bottle.

4. Apply the body oil once you've toweled off after a shower or bath. This will allow the oils to penetrate deeply into the skin. Do not use before bed, as this blend is energizing.

5. Enjoy and feel vital and alive!

# alive and focused roller

Feeling tired? Sluggish? Distracted? Stressed? This blend promotes focus, increases motivation, boosts energy, and reduces stress to make you feel alive and focused. The roll-on application is convenient to bring anywhere and use any time. I love to use this mid-afternoon if I lose my ambition, focus, or energy.

1 (10-milliliter)
roll-on bottle

4 plastic pipettes

2 drops ginger oil

3 drops grapefruit oil

3 drops lemon oil

10 milliliters carrier oil
of your choice

▸ Makes: 10 milliliters

▸ Topical use

▸ Safe for ages 5+

⚠ Do not use for
12 hours before being
in direct sunlight or
a tanning bed.

1. Using the plastic pipettes, add the essential oils to the 10-milliliter roll-on bottle. Twist the cap on and gently swirl the bottle for about 1 minute.

2. Add the carrier oil, cover, and gently swirl the bottle for about 2 minutes to blend. Label the bottle.

3. Roll onto the bottoms of your feet, onto the back of your neck, over your kidneys, and onto your wrists so you can inhale anytime you need.

4. Enjoy and feel alive and focused!

# energize roller

Energy is a necessity! Without energy, your body cannot function. This blend is for the occasional low-energy days after a late night out or poor night's sleep, during a change in diet, or while decreasing caffeine intake. If you are dealing with chronic fatigue, there is an underlying cause and you should see a physician or holistic practitioner. This blend is helpful for chronic fatigue, but it won't fix the underlying cause.

1 (10-milliliter)
roll-on bottle

4 plastic pipettes

4 drops grapefruit oil

3 drops juniper oil

1 drop peppermint oil

10 milliliters carrier oil
of your choice

▸ Makes: 10 milliliters

▸ Topical use

▸ Safe for ages 5+

⚠ Do not use for
12 hours before being
in direct sunlight or
a tanning bed.

1. Using the plastic pipettes, add the essential oils to the 10-milliliter roll-on bottle. Twist the cap on and gently swirl the bottle for about 1 minute.

2. Add the carrier oil, cover, and gently swirl the bottle for about 2 minutes to blend. Label the bottle.

3. Roll onto the bottoms of your feet, onto the back of your neck, over your kidneys, and onto your wrists so you can inhale anytime you need.

4. Enjoy and energize!

# sore muscle relief rub

This rub is great for any time you are experiencing sore and tight muscles. You can use it after exercising or if you sleep in a strange position and wake up with a sore neck. I love to massage this onto my trapezius muscles after a long day sitting at a computer, allowing my shoulders and neck to relax and the tension to melt away—plus it smells amazing and the peppermint oil gives you a cooling sensation.

1 (2-ounce) plastic squeeze bottle with flip top

4 plastic pipettes

15 drops ginger oil

16 drops juniper oil

25 drops lavender oil

16 drops peppermint oil

2 ounces unscented lotion

▸ Makes: 2 ounces

▸ Topical use

▸ Safe for ages 10+

1. Using the plastic pipettes, add the essential oils to a small glass bowl and stir to mix them together.

2. Add the unscented lotion to the bowl and stir until combined. This may take a couple of minutes.

3. Use a spoon to pour the lotion and oil mixture into the 2-ounce squeeze bottle. Label the bottle.

4. Rub and massage this blend into sore and tight muscles.

5. Enjoy and feel relief!

# clear and protect spritzer

The "clear and protect" name for this blend refers to clearing your energy, resetting your chakras, promoting relaxation, and protecting your energy. Throughout the day, you tend to take on the energy of anyone you come in contact with. This spritzer will help you separate your energy from other people's energy. I like to think of it as a bubble. You are in your bubble, which is filled with your energy. When a negative person comes around you, your bubble keeps that negative energy out.

1 (2-ounce) spray bottle

3 plastic pipettes

15 drops ginger oil

15 drops lavender oil

18 drops lemon oil

2 ounces water

▸ Makes: 2 ounces

▸ Indirect inhalation, topical use

▸ Safe for ages 5+

⚠ Do not use for 12 hours before being in direct sunlight or a tanning bed.

1. Using the plastic pipettes, add the essential oils to the 2-ounce spray bottle.

2. Twist the cap on and swirl the bottle for about 1 minute.

3. Remove the cap and add water.

4. Twist the cap back on and swirl for about 2 minutes. Label the bottle.

5. Shake before use and spritz as needed. This can be used as a body or room spritzer. It can be used first thing in the morning or during the day when you feel other people's energy isn't serving you.

6. Enjoy and feel cleared and protected!

# instant energy body wash

This is an affordable body wash with clean ingredients and energizing essential oils. The plastic foaming dispenser makes it easy to use in the shower. I use this body wash every morning to start my day with energy and positivity. Vegetable glycerin moisturizes the skin, but this recipe works equally well without it, so don't worry if you are unable to find it.

1 (12-ounce) plastic foaming dispenser

3 plastic pipettes

18 drops grapefruit oil

22 drops lemon oil

8 drops peppermint oil

⅓ cup liquid castile soap

⅓ cup honey

⅓ cup carrier oil of your choice

1 tablespoon vegetable glycerin (optional)

▸ Makes: 12 ounces

▸ Topical use

▸ Safe for ages 5+

⚠ Do not use for 12 hours before being in direct sunlight or a tanning bed.

1. Using the plastic pipettes, add the essential oils to the 12-ounce plastic foaming dispenser. Twist the cap on and swirl the bottle gently for about 1 minute.

2. Remove the cap and add the castile soap, honey, carrier oil, and glycerin.

3. Twist the cap on and swirl the bottle gently for about 2 minutes to combine. Label the bottle.

4. Dispense the soap into your hands or onto a washcloth or loofa. Lather over wet skin and rinse off.

5. Enjoy and have instant energy!

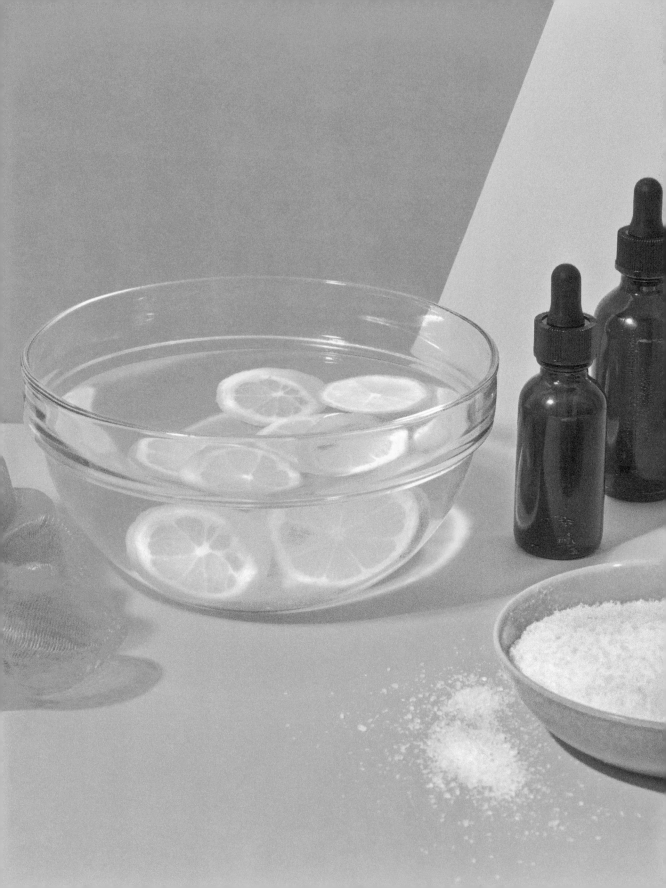

# detox

# detoxifying diffuser blend

Your body accumulates toxins from the food you eat, the environment, the air, and the products you put on your skin. It is impossible to live toxin-free because some things are out of your control; however, you can control the things you put in and on your body. This diffuser blend helps eliminate toxins in the air and in your body. Work on improving the quality of the food you consume, finding clean skincare and haircare products, and diffuse this blend so your body can run efficiently and focus on burning fat instead of eliminating toxins.

1 (10-milliliter) euro dropper bottle

2 plastic pipettes

90 drops juniper oil

120 drops lemon oil

Diffuser

▸ Makes: 10 milliliters (approximately 20 uses)

▸ Indirect inhalation

▸ Safe for all ages

1. Using the plastic pipettes, add the essential oils to the 10-milliliter euro dropper bottle.

2. Reinsert the orifice reducer that came with the bottle, secure the cap, and gently swirl the bottle for about 1 minute. Label the bottle.

3. Add 8 to 12 drops to your diffuser and diffuse in 30-minute increments.

4. Enjoy and detox!

# anti-cellulite massage oil

This massage oil works to promote circulation, which helps reduce the appearance of cellulite and tighten the skin. This blend can also be applied preventively to areas where cellulite is common, such as the buttocks, thighs, and hips. This pairs well with the Cellulite Buster Cream on page 77.

1 (2-ounce) glass dropper bottle

3 plastic pipettes

15 drops grapefruit oil

20 drops juniper oil

20 drops lavender oil

2 ounces carrier oil of your choice (sesame oil is recommended)

▸ Makes: 2 ounces

▸ Topical use

▸ Safe for ages 5+

⚠ Do not use for 12 hours before being in direct sunlight or a tanning bed.

1. Using the plastic pipettes, add the essential oils to the 2-ounce glass dropper bottle.

2. Twist the cap on and gently swirl the bottle for about 1 minute.

3. Add the carrier oil, cover, and gently swirl the bottle for about 2 minutes to blend. Label the bottle.

4. Massage into skin where cellulite is present. This can also be used to prevent cellulite by massaging into areas of concern, such as buttocks, thighs, and hips.

5. Enjoy and smooth your skin!

# fat burning massage oil

This fat-burning blend promotes healthy digestion, boosts metabolism, and eliminates toxins. It won't cause weight loss, but with a healthy diet, exercise, and a positive attitude, it can help you lose inches. I love to massage this onto my abdomen in a clockwise direction daily to supplement my healthy lifestyle, promote weight loss, and regulate digestion.

1 (2-ounce) glass dropper bottle

3 plastic pipettes

20 drops ginger oil

36 drops grapefruit oil

8 drops peppermint oil

2 ounces carrier oil of your choice

▸ Makes: 2 ounces

▸ Topical use

▸ Safe for ages 5+

⚠ Do not use for 12 hours before being in direct sunlight or a tanning bed.

1. Using the plastic pipettes, add the essential oils to the 2-ounce glass dropper bottle.

2. Twist the cap on and gently swirl the bottle for about 1 minute.

3. Add the carrier oil, cover, and gently swirl the bottle for about 2 minutes to blend. Label the bottle.

4. Massage into areas where fat is accumulating. If you can reach or have someone else massage the oil blend onto your back, that is also beneficial.

5. Enjoy and burn some fat!

# liver health massage oil

The liver is an important organ that helps metabolize fat, eliminate toxins, and boost energy. When it is healthy, you are more likely to lose weight. A lifestyle including high-fat foods and high levels of stress can negatively affect liver health. Using this massage oil will help boost liver health, but it is also important to reduce the amount of processed foods, meat, and dairy consumed, and to manage stress levels. (Aromatherapy significantly helps reduce stress levels naturally; see chapter 8 for helpful stress-relieving recipes.)

1 (2-ounce) glass dropper bottle

3 plastic pipettes

10 drops ginger oil

18 drops grapefruit oil

20 drops lemon oil

2 ounces carrier oil of your choice

▸ Makes: 2 ounces

▸ Topical use

▸ Safe for ages 5+

⚠ Do not use for 12 hours before being in direct sunlight or a tanning bed.

1. Using the plastic pipettes, add the essential oils to the 2-ounce glass dropper bottle.

2. Twist the cap on and gently swirl the bottle for about 1 minute.

3. Add the carrier oil, cover, and gently swirl the bottle for about 2 minutes to blend. Label the bottle.

4. Massage below the ribs and onto the abdomen in a clockwise motion. If you can reach or have someone else massage the oil blend onto your mid-back, that is also beneficial.

5. Enjoy and improve your liver health!

# detox roller

This blend helps remove toxins from the liver, kidneys, intestines, and lymphatic system. I occasionally have meals that don't align with my typical healthy diet. When this happens, I tend to feel sluggish and fatigued. This blend naturally boosts energy and promotes digestion and lymphatic drainage, which is why I keep it in my purse for just those occasions.

**1 (10-milliliter) roll-on bottle**

**4 plastic pipettes**

**3 drops grapefruit oil**

**3 drops juniper oil**

**2 drops peppermint oil**

**10 milliliters carrier oil of your choice**

▸ Makes: 10 milliliters

▸ Topical use

▸ Safe for ages 5+

⚠ Do not use for 12 hours before being in direct sunlight or a tanning bed.

1. Using the plastic pipettes, add the essential oils to the 10-milliliter roll-on bottle. Twist the cap on and gently swirl the bottle for about 1 minute.

2. Add the carrier oil, cover, and gently swirl the bottle for about 2 minutes to blend. Label the bottle.

3. Roll onto the bottoms of your feet, onto your abdomen in a clockwise motion, and onto your wrists so you can inhale anytime you want.

4. Enjoy and detoxify your body!

# cellulite buster cream

Cellulite is more prevalent in women than in men, and it becomes more common as you age. Cellulite can be frustrating and may affect your confidence, but it's important to remember that the appearance of cellulite does not mean a person is overweight or out of shape. Improving circulation can help reduce the appearance of cellulite, and dry brushing is a great way to improve circulation. (Dry brushing is when you use a brush with firm bristles directly on the skin to increase blood flow to the skin, remove dead skin cells, reduce the appearance of cellulite, and promote detoxification. Brush the skin in a circular motion starting with the hands and feet, and always brush toward the heart.) This blend is most effective when you dry brush first, take a warm shower or bath, and then massage this cream into the affected areas.

1 (8-ounce) Mason jar

3 plastic pipettes

22 drops fennel oil

20 drops lavender oil

30 drops lemon oil

¼ cup (2 ounces) coconut oil

▶ Makes: 2 ounces

▶ Topical use

▶ Safe for ages 5+

⚠ Do not use for 12 hours before being in direct sunlight or a tanning bed. Avoid use during pregnancy, while breastfeeding, and if you have an estrogen-dependent cancer or endometriosis.

1. Using the plastic pipettes, add the essential oils to a small glass bowl and stir to mix them together.

2. Add the coconut oil and mix until it is a smooth, creamy texture. It is easiest to use a hand mixer, but a whisk will work, too.

3. Transfer the mixture to the Mason jar. Label the jar.

4. Rub and massage this blend into areas where cellulite is present. This can also be used to prevent cellulite by massaging into areas of concern such as buttocks, thighs, and hips.

5. Enjoy and reduce the appearance of cellulite!

# stretch mark remover cream

Stretch marks can appear quickly with sudden weight gain or loss, but don't let them get you down! When you lose the weight, they will be less noticeable—and when you use this cream consistently, they will fade more and more.

1 (8-ounce) Mason jar

3 plastic pipettes

30 drops grapefruit oil

24 drops lavender oil

18 drops patchouli oil

¼ cup (2 ounces) coconut oil

▶ Makes: 2 ounces

▶ Topical use

▶ Safe for ages 5+

⚠ Do not use for 12 hours before being in direct sunlight or a tanning bed.

1. Using the plastic pipettes, add the essential oils to a small glass bowl and stir to mix them together.

2. Add the coconut oil and mix until it is a smooth, creamy texture. It is easiest to use a hand mixer, but a whisk will work, too.

3. Transfer the mixture to the Mason jar. Label the jar.

4. Rub and massage this blend into areas where stretch marks are present. This can also be used to prevent stretch marks by massaging into areas of concern such as abdomen, buttocks, thighs, hips, and breasts.

5. Enjoy and remove those stretch marks!

# cleanse and restore bath soak

Taking the time to regularly clear your thoughts and restore your energy is an important component of any weight loss process. This bath soak is like a reset button for the body. Himalayan salt is great for cleansing your body of toxins and clearing your respiratory system. It can be used morning, day, or night, as it is calming and clearing. I love to make large batches of this recipe to store in Mason jars for easy later use.

1 (8-ounce) Mason jar

3 plastic pipettes

2 drops ginger oil

2 drops juniper oil

5 drops lavender oil

1 cup Himalayan salt (texture can be coarse or fine)

▸ Makes: 1 cup (1 use)

▸ Topical use

▸ Safe for ages 5+

1. Using the plastic pipettes, add the essential oils to a small glass bowl and stir to mix them together.

2. Add the Himalayan salt and stir to combine.

3. If you prefer to store this for future use, pour into a Mason jar and label the jar.

4. When you are ready to use it, pour the salt mixture into the bathtub and fill with warm water.

5. Enjoy and feel your body cleanse and restore!

# purify bath salt

Epsom salt is known for flushing toxins from the body and reducing inflammation. The essential oils in this blend clear, protect, ground, calm, motivate, and energize. Throughout your weight loss journey, it is important to purify and cleanse your body and mind. While using this bath salt, try saying affirmations like, "I am positive and protected. I let go of expectations. My body and mind support me. I am healthy, happy, and successful."

1 (8-ounce) Mason jar

3 plastic pipettes

3 drops ginger oil

6 drops lavender oil

3 drops lemon oil

1 cup Epsom salt (texture can be coarse or fine)

▸ Makes: 1 cup (1 use)

▸ Topical use

▸ Safe for ages 5+

⚠ Do not use for 12 hours before being in direct sunlight or a tanning bed.

1. Using the plastic pipettes, add the essential oils to a small glass bowl and stir to mix them together.

2. Add the Epsom salt and stir to combine.

3. If you prefer to store this for future use, pour into a Mason jar and label the jar.

4. When you are ready to use it, pour the salt mixture into the bathtub and fill with warm water.

5. Enjoy and purify your body and mind!

# detox scrub

Body scrubs are amazing for exfoliating, reducing impurities, and pulling toxins out of the body. Plus, they leave your skin feeling soft, smooth, rejuvenated, and refreshed! I enjoy using this scrub once or twice a week so that my skin feels amazing and my body can eliminate toxins. As you use this scrub, imagine the toxins being pulled from your body and your energy being renewed. Remember to apply a body oil or moisturizer after using a scrub to replenish your skin.

1 (8-ounce) Mason jar

3 plastic pipettes

13 drops fennel oil

19 drops juniper oil

32 drops lemon oil

6 ounces Epsom salt (fine texture)

¼ cup (2 ounces) almond or sunflower oil

▸ Makes: 1 cup

▸ Topical use

▸ Safe for ages 5+

⚠ Do not use for 12 hours before being in direct sunlight or a tanning bed. Avoid use during pregnancy, while breastfeeding, and if you have an estrogen-dependent cancer or endometriosis.

1. Using the plastic pipettes, add the essential oils to an 8-ounce Mason jar.

2. Twist the cap on and swirl gently for about 1 minute.

3. Add the carrier oil, cover, and gently swirl the bottle for about 2 minutes to blend.

4. Gradually stir the salt into the oil mixture. Label the bottle.

5. Stir before each use. Massage into wet skin. Rinse off and make sure to replenish your skin afterward by moisturizing with a body oil or cream.

6. Enjoy and pull out the toxins!

# stimulating scrub for cellulite

Scrubs promote circulation and lymphatic drainage, which can help reduce the appearance of cellulite and tighten the skin. This scrub can be used on the whole body, or you can focus on areas where cellulite is present or common, such as the buttocks, thighs, and hips. After exfoliating, it is important to moisturize with a body oil or cream. Using the Cellulite Buster Cream (page 77) after this scrub will improve results.

1 (8-ounce) Mason jar

3 plastic pipettes

23 drops grapefruit oil

17 drops juniper oil

23 drops lemon oil

6 ounces Epsom salt (fine texture)

¼ cup (2 ounces) almond or sunflower oil

▸ Makes: 1 cup

▸ Topical use

▸ Safe for ages 5+

⚠ Do not use for 12 hours before being in direct sunlight or a tanning bed

1. Using the plastic pipettes, add the essential oils to an 8-ounce Mason jar.

2. Twist the cap on and swirl gently for about 1 minute.

3. Add the carrier oil, cover, and gently swirl the bottle for about 2 minutes to blend.

4. Gradually stir the salt into the oil mixture. Label the bottle.

5. Stir before each use. Massage into wet skin where cellulite is present. This can also be used to prevent cellulite by massaging into areas of concern such as buttocks, thighs, and hips. Rinse off and make sure to replenish your skin afterward by moisturizing with a body oil or cream.

6. Enjoy and promote circulation!

# smoothing and firming cellulite body wrap

If you have cellulite or loose skin, or are looking to burn fat, this body wrap is for you! Body wraps are perfect for increasing circulation, eliminating toxins, and smoothing and tightening the skin. They are most effective after a hot shower as heat opens your pores for easy absorption of the oil blend. I cannot stress enough how important it is to drink water before, during, and after your wrap to stay hydrated.

1 (2-ounce) glass dropper bottle

3 plastic pipettes

22 drops fennel oil

30 drops grapefruit oil

20 drops lemon oil

2 ounces carrier oil of your choice (sesame oil is recommended)

▸ Makes: 2 ounces

▸ Topical use

▸ Safe for ages 5+

⚠ Do not use for 12 hours before being in direct sunlight or a tanning bed. Avoid use during pregnancy, while breastfeeding, or if you have an estrogen-dependent cancer or endometriosis.

1. Using the plastic pipettes, add the essential oils to the 2-ounce glass dropper bottle.

2. Twist the cap on and gently swirl the bottle for about 1 minute.

3. Add the carrier oil, cover, and gently swirl the bottle for about 2 minutes to blend. Label the bottle.

4. Massage the oil blend into your waist, thighs, buttocks, or other areas where cellulite is present. Place a lightweight fabric (muslin or an old T-shirt) on the area, then wrap with about 5 layers of plastic wrap to hold the fabric in place. Leave the wrap on for 1 hour. Be sure to drink water before, during, and after using this wrap.

5. Enjoy and smooth and firm your skin!

# digestion

# anti-nausea inhaler

Nausea can make you very uncomfortable and uneasy, and inhaling essential oils can significantly reduce nausea. The essential oils in this blend help settle the stomach, calm the nervous system, clear your mind, aid digestion, and reduce bloating. While using the inhaler, focus on the now and repeat affirmations such as, "I am grounded. I am safe. I am calm. I trust the process of life."

**Blank inhaler**

**3 plastic pipettes**

**13 drops ginger oil**

**12 drops lavender oil**

**5 drops peppermint oil**

▸ Makes: 1 inhaler

▸ Direct inhalation

▸ Safe for ages 5+

1. Using the plastic pipettes, mix the essential oils in a small glass bowl.

2. Remove the cover on the inhaler tube. Using tweezers, place the wick in the bowl of essential oils and move it around until the essential oils are absorbed.

3. Use tweezers to place the moistened wick back in the inhaler tube.

4. Put the cover back on to secure the wick. Label the inhaler.

5. Twist off the cap and inhale the aroma for 2 to 5 minutes at a time.

6. Enjoy and be nausea-free!

# anti-inflammatory massage oil

Inflammation can negatively affect every organ. This oil can be used for full body massages to reduce inflammation and tension throughout the body; localized massages where you feel tension, soreness, and pain; abdominal massages to reduce inflammation in the gut; and post-workout massages to help prevent sore muscles the following day.

1 (2-ounce) glass dropper bottle

3 plastic pipettes

13 drops ginger oil

20 drops lavender oil

5 drops peppermint oil

2 ounces carrier oil of your choice

▸ Makes: 2 ounces

▸ Topical use

▸ Safe for ages 5+

1. Using the plastic pipettes, add the essential oils to the 2-ounce glass dropper bottle.

2. Twist the cap on and gently swirl the bottle for about 1 minute.

3. Add the carrier oil, cover, and gently swirl the bottle for about 2 minutes to blend. Label the bottle.

4. Rub and massage this blend into painful, sore, or tight muscles. If you can reach or have someone else massage the oil blend into your back, that is also beneficial.

5. Enjoy and reduce inflammation in your body!

# bloat-less massage oil

That bloated sensation, when your stomach feels uncomfortably full and swollen, is often due to diet. It is important to learn which foods your body is reacting to and then limit them. When you do feel bloated and full, however, this blend can be massaged onto the abdomen to promote healthy digestion and reduce bloat. It also helps relieve gas, which commonly goes hand in hand with bloating.

1 (2-ounce) glass dropper bottle

3 plastic pipettes

17 drops fennel oil

23 drops ginger oil

8 drops peppermint oil

¼ cup (2 ounces) carrier oil of your choice

▸ Makes: 2 ounces

▸ Topical use

▸ Safe for ages 5+

⚠ Avoid use during pregnancy, while breastfeeding, and if you have an estrogen-dependent cancer or endometriosis.

1. Using the plastic pipettes, add the essential oils to the 2-ounce glass dropper bottle.

2. Twist the cap on and gently swirl the bottle for about 1 minute.

3. Add the carrier oil, cover, and gently swirl the bottle for about 2 minutes to blend. Label the bottle.

4. Massage into the abdomen to reduce bloat and regulate digestion. Massage in a clockwise direction for constipation and counterclockwise for diarrhea.

5. Enjoy and bloat less!

# constipation relief massage oil

Constipation can cause weight gain, stomach pain, cramping, and discomfort. Massaging this blend into the abdomen in a clockwise direction can be very helpful. Why clockwise? Because that is the natural direction of your digestive system. It is also important to make sure you are getting enough fiber in your diet and that you are exercising and moving your body.

1 (2-ounce) glass dropper bottle

3 plastic pipettes

24 drops fennel oil

24 drops ginger oil

24 drops lemon oil

2 ounces carrier oil of your choice

▸ Makes: 2 ounces

▸ Topical use

▸ Safe for ages 5+

⚠ Do not use for 12 hours before being in direct sunlight or a tanning bed. Avoid use during pregnancy, while breastfeeding, and if you have an estrogen-dependent cancer or endometriosis.

1. Using the plastic pipettes, add the essential oils to the 2-ounce glass dropper bottle.

2. Twist the cap on and gently swirl the bottle for about 1 minute.

3. Add the carrier oil, cover, and gently swirl the bottle for about 2 minutes to blend. Label the bottle.

4. Massage into the abdomen in a clockwise direction to relieve constipation and regulate digestion.

5. Enjoy and feel relief!

# regulate digestion massage oil

Throughout your weight loss journey, you will likely experiment with different foods and types of exercise to find the formula that works best for you. Digestion is the process of absorbing nutrients from the food you eat and eliminating what your body doesn't need. The more regular your digestion is, the healthier you will be. Digestion can be worsened or improved by diet, and learning what's best for your body can take time. As you experiment, this massage oil can be used to promote regular, healthy digestion.

1 (2-ounce) glass dropper bottle

3 plastic pipettes

30 drops lemon oil

18 drops peppermint oil

2 ounces carrier oil of your choice

▸ Makes: 2 ounces

▸ Topical use

▸ Safe for ages 5+

⚠ Do not use for 12 hours before being in direct sunlight or a tanning bed.

1. Using the plastic pipettes, add the essential oils to the 2-ounce glass dropper bottle.

2. Twist the cap on and gently swirl the bottle for about 1 minute.

3. Add the carrier oil, cover, and gently swirl the bottle for about 2 minutes to blend. Label the bottle.

4. Massage into the abdomen to regulate digestion. Massage in a clockwise direction for constipation and counterclockwise for diarrhea.

5. Enjoy and be regular!

# stomach cramp–ease massage oil

When the stomach lining is inflamed, you'll feel stomach cramps. It is important to reduce consumption of inflammatory foods for optimal absorption of nutrients, which will also help regulate digestion and reduce inflammation in the gut. When you experience stomach cramping, massage this blend into the abdomen to experience relief and promote healthy digestion.

**1 (2-ounce) glass dropper bottle**

**3 plastic pipettes**

**20 drops fennel oil**

**20 drops juniper oil**

**24 drops lavender oil**

**2 ounces carrier oil of your choice**

▸ Makes: 2 ounces

▸ Topical use

▸ Safe for ages 5+

⚠ Avoid use during pregnancy, while breastfeeding, and if you have an estrogen-dependent cancer or endometriosis.

1. Using the plastic pipettes, add the essential oils to the 2-ounce glass dropper bottle.

2. Twist the cap on and gently swirl the bottle for about 1 minute.

3. Add the carrier oil, cover, and gently swirl the bottle for about 2 minutes to blend. Label the bottle.

4. Massage into the abdomen to relieve digestive cramping and regulate digestion. Massage in a clockwise direction for constipation and counterclockwise for diarrhea.

5. Enjoy and ease the cramps!

# digest-ease roller

Sometimes digestive concerns show up out of the blue, which is why I've put this blend in a roll-on bottle: It's easy to apply on the go. It's a versatile blend that helps relieve stomach cramping, gas, constipation, diarrhea, discomfort, nausea, heartburn, and acid reflux. Store it in your purse or backpack and use it whenever you need it.

**1 (10-milliliter) roll-on bottle**

**4 plastic pipettes**

**3 drops fennel oil**

**3 drops juniper oil**

**2 drops lemon oil**

**10 milliliters carrier oil of your choice**

▸ Makes: 10 milliliters

▸ Topical use

▸ Safe for ages 5+

⚠ Do not use for 12 hours before being in direct sunlight or a tanning bed. Avoid use during pregnancy, while breastfeeding, and if you have an estrogen-dependent cancer or endometriosis.

1. Using the plastic pipettes, add the essential oils to the 10-milliliter roll-on bottle. Twist the cap on and gently swirl the bottle for about 1 minute.

2. Add the carrier oil, cover, and gently swirl the bottle for about 2 minutes to blend. Label the bottle.

3. Roll onto the abdomen in a clockwise motion and onto the bottoms of your feet to regulate digestion.

4. Enjoy and ease digestion!

# gas relief roller

Gas can cause significant stomach pain and cramping if you hold it in. Remember, passing gas is a regular bodily function, and everyone does it! This blend can be used topically on the abdomen and bottoms of your feet to relieve gas. It helps to learn what foods might be causing your excess gas so you can avoid or reduce consumption in the future.

1 (10-milliliter) roll-on bottle

4 plastic pipettes

3 drops fennel oil

4 drops ginger oil

1 drop juniper oil

10 milliliters carrier oil of your choice

▶ Makes: 10 milliliters

▶ Topical use

▶ Safe for ages 5+

⚠ Avoid use during pregnancy, while breastfeeding, and if you have an estrogen-dependent cancer or endometriosis.

1. Using the plastic pipettes, add the essential oils to the 10-milliliter roll-on bottle. Twist the cap on and gently swirl the bottle for about 1 minute.

2. Add the carrier oil, cover, and gently swirl the bottle for about 2 minutes to blend. Label the bottle.

3. Roll onto the abdomen in a clockwise motion and onto the bottoms of your feet to release gas and reduce bloating.

4. Enjoy and let it go!

# gut healing roller

Healthy changes to your diet can help heal your gut and promote regular elimination. Foods that support gut healing include fermented vegetables, raw vegetables, fruits, nuts, and seeds. Talk to your physician or holistic practitioner about supplements and diets that support gut health. This gut healing roller is great for general digestive concerns such as constipation, diarrhea, gas, and cramping.

1 (10-milliliter) roll-on bottle

4 plastic pipettes

2 drops ginger oil

3 drops lemon oil

3 drops peppermint oil

10 milliliters carrier oil of your choice

▸ Makes: 10 milliliters

▸ Topical use

▸ Safe for ages 5+

⚠ Do not use for 12 hours before being in direct sunlight or a tanning bed.

1. Using the plastic pipettes, add the essential oils to the 10-milliliter roll-on bottle. Twist the cap on and gently swirl the bottle for about 1 minute.

2. Add the carrier oil, cover, and gently swirl the bottle for about 2 minutes to blend. Label the bottle.

3. Roll onto the abdomen in a clockwise motion and onto the bottoms of your feet to heal the gut and improve gut health.

4. Enjoy and heal your gut!

# heartburn relief roller

Heartburn is when you experience a burning sensation in your chest and/
or throat, commonly triggered by foods that are fatty, spicy, or salty, as
well as alcohol, caffeine, dairy, carbonated sodas, and more. The foods
that cause heartburn can vary from person to person. This blend helps
relieve the general symptoms of heartburn. If heartburn is occurring
regularly and isn't linked to a specific food, please see your physician or
holistic practitioner.

1 (10-milliliter)
roll-on bottle

4 plastic pipettes

3 drops ginger oil

2 drops lavender oil

3 drops lemon oil

10 milliliters carrier oil
of your choice

▸ Makes: 10 milliliters

▸ Topical use

▸ Safe for ages 5+

⚠ Do not use for
12 hours before being
in direct sunlight or
a tanning bed.

1. Using the plastic pipettes, add the essential oils to the
   10-milliliter roll-on bottle. Twist the cap on and gently swirl
   the bottle for about 1 minute.

2. Add the carrier oil, cover, and gently swirl the bottle for
   about 2 minutes to blend. Label the bottle.

3. Roll onto the bottoms of your feet, onto your abdomen in
   a clockwise motion, and onto your wrists so you can inhale
   anytime you need.

4. Enjoy and find relief!

# nervous tummy roller

Have you ever been nervous before a meeting, speech, or doctor's appointment and felt uneasy in your stomach? Anxiety and nervousness can affect your stomach and digestion. Using this roller on your feet, abdomen, and wrists helps calm your stomach and mind. Simultaneously, try to focus on the present moment rather than worrying about the future—pay attention to your breathing and the present moment.

1 (10-milliliter)
roll-on bottle

4 plastic pipettes

3 drops ginger oil

1 drop grapefruit oil

4 drops lavender oil

10 milliliters carrier oil
of your choice

▶ Makes: 10 milliliters

▶ Topical use

▶ Safe for ages 5+

⚠ Do not use for
12 hours before being
in direct sunlight or
a tanning bed.

1. Using the plastic pipettes, add the essential oils to the 10-milliliter roll-on bottle. Twist the cap on and gently swirl the bottle for about 1 minute.

2. Add the carrier oil, cover, and gently swirl the bottle for about 2 minutes to blend. Label the bottle.

3. Roll onto the bottoms of your feet, onto your abdomen in a clockwise motion, and onto your wrists so you can inhale anytime you need.

4. Enjoy and release the nervous feeling!

# acid reflux rub

Acid reflux and heartburn are uncomfortable burning sensations in the chest and throat. It can be difficult to deal with, especially when you are away from home. The more you focus on it, the more uncomfortable you will feel. Use this rub on your abdomen and your chest to help reduce symptoms, and then find something else to focus on. Focus on your breath, the cold air flowing in your nostrils, and the warm air flowing out of your nostrils. Go grab a book, take a bath, or repeat positive affirmations. Whatever you do, try to take your mind off the acid reflux.

1 (8-ounce) Mason jar

3 plastic pipettes

12 drops lavender oil

21 drops lemon oil

15 drops peppermint oil

¼ cup (2 ounces) coconut oil

▶ Makes: 2 ounces

▶ Topical use

▶ Safe for ages 5+

⚠ Do not use for 12 hours before being in direct sunlight or a tanning bed.

1. Using the plastic pipettes, add the essential oils to a small glass bowl and stir to mix them together.

2. Add the coconut oil and mix. It is easiest to use a hand mixer, but a whisk will work, too.

3. Transfer the mixture to the Mason jar. Label the jar.

4. Massage into the abdomen in a clockwise direction to relieve acid reflux. This blend can also be massaged into the chest.

5. Enjoy, breathe, and be in the present moment!

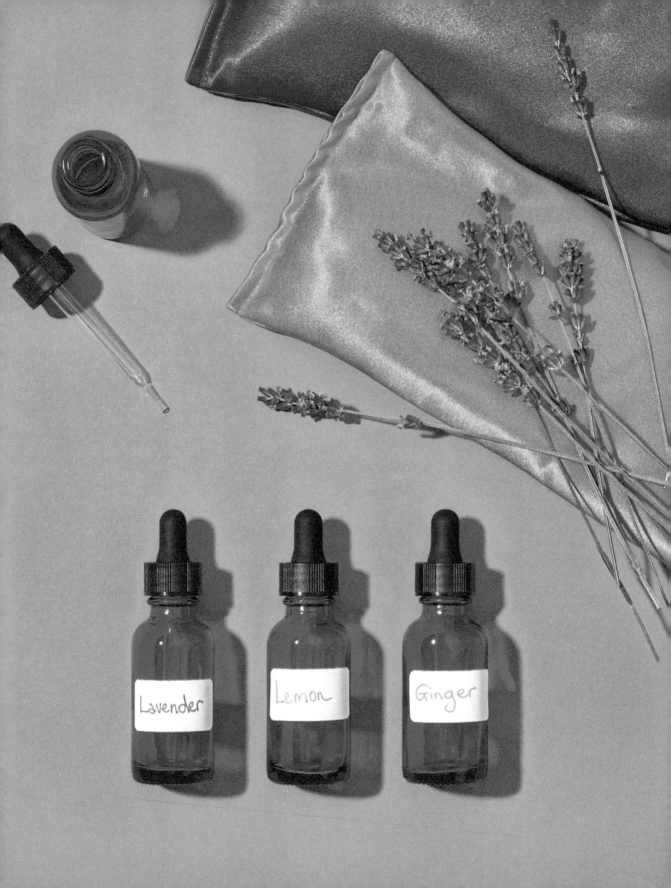

# sleep & calm

# mental clarity in a bottle diffuser blend

Challenges in life are inevitable. Having a clear mind is important, especially when you need to make a decision. This blend helps you get through life's challenges with mental clarity. Anytime I feel like my judgment is clouded, I diffuse this blend for clarity and support. This blend is also uplifting, to leave you feeling happy, content, and confident in your decisions.

1 (10-milliliter) euro dropper bottle

3 plastic pipettes

70 drops ginger oil

120 drops lemon oil

20 drops peppermint oil

Diffuser

▸ Makes: 10 milliliters (approximately 20 uses)

▸ Indirect inhalation

▸ Safe for 5+

1. Using the plastic pipettes, add the essential oils to the 10-milliliter euro dropper bottle.

2. Reinsert the orifice reducer that came with the bottle, secure the cap, and gently swirl the bottle for about 1 minute. Label the bottle.

3. Add 8 to 12 drops to your diffuser and diffuse in 30-minute increments.

4. Enjoy and find clarity!

# emotion balance diffuser blend

Emotions vary day to day and sometimes even minute to minute. In life, it is important to feel balanced physically, emotionally, and mentally. This blend will help you do just that, as well as help you center yourself when you're having an off day. If I am feeling sad, I will diffuse this blend to add happiness and joy into my life.

1 (10-milliliter) euro dropper bottle

3 plastic pipettes

30 drops fennel oil

100 drops grapefruit oil

80 drops juniper oil

Diffuser

▸ Makes: 10 milliliters (approximately 20 uses)

▸ Indirect inhalation

▸ Safe for ages 5+

⚠ Avoid use during pregnancy, while breastfeeding, and if you have an estrogen-dependent cancer or endometriosis.

1. Using the plastic pipettes, add the essential oils to the 10-milliliter euro dropper bottle.

2. Reinsert the orifice reducer that came with the bottle, secure the cap, and gently swirl the bottle for about 1 minute. Label the bottle.

3. Add 8 to 12 drops to your diffuser and diffuse in 30-minute increments.

4. Enjoy and feel balanced!

# sleep deeply diffuser blend

Proper sleep is essential, especially while you're losing weight. Increased appetite, frequent cravings, low energy, sluggish metabolism, forgetfulness, and moodiness can be signs of not enough sleep or of poor-quality sleep. To improve sleep quality, turn off electronics at least an hour before going to bed, go to sleep and wake up at consistent times, discontinue caffeine in the evening, avoid alcohol, and diffuse this blend.

1 (10-milliliter) euro dropper bottle

3 plastic pipettes

120 drops lavender oil

70 drops patchouli oil

20 drops vetiver oil

Diffuser

▸ Makes: 10 milliliters (approximately 20 uses)

▸ Indirect inhalation

▸ Safe for all ages

1. Using the plastic pipettes, add the essential oils to the 10-milliliter euro dropper bottle.

2. Reinsert the orifice reducer that came with the bottle, secure the cap, and gently swirl the bottle for about 1 minute. Label the bottle.

3. Add 8 to 12 drops to your diffuser and diffuse in 30-minute increments.

4. Enjoy and sleep deeply!

# find inner peace inhaler

At times, your weight loss journey might feel overwhelming, chaotic, and challenging. This inhaler works to promote inner peace to leave you feeling content, calm, and serene. While using this inhaler, breathe deeply, focus on your progress, be patient, slow down, and let go of the past, negative thoughts, and emotions. You *can* and *will* get through this journey—and you will learn so much about your mind and body along the way.

**Blank inhaler**

**3 plastic pipettes**

**12 drops lemon oil**

**12 drops lavender oil**

**6 drops patchouli oil**

▸ Makes: 1 inhaler

▸ Direct inhalation

▸ Safe for all ages

1. Using the plastic pipettes, mix the essential oils in a small glass bowl.

2. Remove the cover on the inhaler tube. Using tweezers, place the wick in the bowl of essential oils and move it around until the essential oils are absorbed.

3. Use tweezers to place the moistened wick back in the inhaler tube.

4. Put the cover back on to secure the wick. Label the inhaler.

5. Twist off the cap and inhale the aroma for 2 to 5 minutes at a time.

6. Enjoy and find peace!

# uplifting inhaler

Are you feeling frustrated, sad, angry, or depressed? Have you hit a plateau? Do you feel lost and confused? Negative, unproductive thoughts may arise during your weight loss journey. This inhaler is here to uplift and support you. It will help improve your mood, boost your energy, and promote positive thoughts. Believe in yourself, be gentle and forgiving with yourself, let go of the past, and repeat positive affirmations that relate to your situation. For example, if you feel you have hit a plateau, repeat, "I love and accept myself. I love myself unconditionally. I am proud of myself."

**Blank inhaler**

**3 plastic pipettes**

**6 drops ginger oil**

**13 drops grapefruit oil**

**11 drops lemon oil**

▶ Makes: 1 inhaler

▶ Direct inhalation

▶ Safe for all ages

1. Using the plastic pipettes, mix the essential oils in a small glass bowl.

2. Remove the cover on the inhaler tube. Using tweezers, place the wick in the bowl of essential oils and move it around until the essential oils are absorbed.

3. Use tweezers to place the moistened wick back in the inhaler tube.

4. Put the cover back on to secure the wick. Label the inhaler.

5. Twist off the cap and inhale the aroma for 2 to 5 minutes at a time.

6. Enjoy and be uplifted!

# tranquility massage oil

This massage oil is great for helping you unwind and find tranquility at the end of the day or anytime you are feeling overwhelmed or anxious. Not only is the aroma delightful, but the essential oils also work with your nervous system to help you feel peaceful. This blend can also be used as a body oil. I love to use it after a shower at the end of the day.

**1 (2-ounce) glass dropper bottle**

**3 plastic pipettes**

**25 drops lavender oil**

**13 drops lemon oil**

**10 drops vetiver oil**

**2 ounces carrier oil of your choice**

▸ Makes: 2 ounces

▸ Topical use

▸ Safe for ages 5+

⚠ Do not use for 12 hours before being in direct sunlight or a tanning bed.

1. Using the plastic pipettes, add the essential oils to the 2-ounce glass dropper bottle.

2. Twist the cap on and gently swirl the bottle for about 1 minute.

3. Add the carrier oil, cover, and gently swirl the bottle for about 2 minutes to blend. Label the bottle.

4. Massage into the body, focusing on the neck or wherever you feel tension.

5. Enjoy and be tranquil!

# stress begone roller

Stress can make it difficult to lose weight and can even contribute to weight gain. Managing stress will help curb cravings, prevent overeating, reduce emotional eating, improve metabolism, and decrease fatigue. Try this blend alone or in conjunction with a stress-relieving activity, such as exercise (especially yoga), meditation, progressive muscle relaxation, positive affirmations, deep breathing, dancing, or a relaxing bath.

1 (10-milliliter) roll-on bottle

4 plastic pipettes

1 drop fennel oil

4 drops grapefruit oil

3 drops lavender oil

10 milliliters carrier oil of your choice

▸ Makes: 10 milliliters

▸ Topical use

▸ Safe for ages 5+

⚠ Do not use for 12 hours before being in direct sunlight or a tanning bed. Avoid use during pregnancy, while breastfeeding, and if you have an estrogen-dependent cancer or endometriosis.

1. Using the plastic pipettes, add the essential oils to the 10-milliliter roll-on bottle. Twist the cap on and gently swirl the bottle for about 1 minute.

2. Add the carrier oil, cover, and gently swirl the bottle for about 2 minutes to blend. Label the bottle.

3. Roll onto the bottoms of your feet, onto the back of your neck, over your kidneys, or onto your wrists so you can inhale anytime you need.

4. Enjoy and relieve stress!

# anxiety relief spritzer

Anxiety is especially likely to turn up during times of transition. Transition can be scary, intimidating, and overwhelming. This spritzer naturally calms and supports the nervous system. When I am feeling anxious, I love to spritz this blend on my body while taking deep breaths. I imagine myself as a tree and visualize my roots growing into the earth. I instantly feel grounded, connected, supported, and in tune with my body.

1 (2-ounce) spray bottle

3 plastic pipettes

12 drops ginger oil

18 drops juniper oil

18 drops patchouli oil

2 ounces water

▸ Makes: 2 ounces

▸ Indirect inhalation, topical use

▸ Safe for all ages

1. Using the plastic pipettes, add the essential oils to the 2-ounce spray bottle.

2. Twist the cap on and swirl the bottle for about 1 minute.

3. Remove the cap and add the water.

4. Twist the cap back on and swirl for about 2 minutes. Label the bottle.

5. Shake before use and spritz as needed. This can be used as a body or room spritzer.

6. Enjoy and release the anxiety!

# calming body wash

This body wash will leave you feeling calm, cool, and collected. It helps clear your mind, calm your nervous system, and relax muscles. It isn't overly sedating *or* energizing, so it can be used morning, day, and night. I enjoy using this blend at the end of the day to relax my body and calm my mind so I can fall asleep easily and sleep deeply. Vegetable glycerin moisturizes the skin, but this recipe works equally well without it, so don't worry if you are unable to find it.

1 (12-ounce) plastic foaming dispenser

3 plastic pipettes

16 drops grapefruit oil

12 drops juniper oil

20 drops lavender oil

⅓ cup liquid castile soap

⅓ cup honey

⅓ cup carrier oil of your choice

1 tablespoon vegetable glycerin (optional)

▶ Makes: 12 ounces

▶ Topical use

▶ Safe for ages 5+

⚠ Do not use for 12 hours before being in direct sunlight or a tanning bed.

1. Using the plastic pipettes, add the essential oils to the 12-ounce plastic foaming dispenser. Twist the cap on and swirl the bottle gently for about 1 minute.

2. Remove the cap and add the castile soap, honey, carrier oil, and glycerin (if using).

3. Twist the cap on and swirl the bottle gently for about 2 minutes to combine. Label the bottle.

4. Dispense the soap into your hands, or onto a washcloth or loofa. Lather over wet skin and rinse off.

5. Enjoy and be calm!

# soak away the day bath salt

Your body benefits from relaxing and restoring at the end of the day. The essential oils in this blend will promote relaxation of the body and mind while the Himalayan salt works to improve circulation, soothe muscle aches and tension, and detoxify the body. When you're in the bath, focus on deep breathing. With each inhale, think of something you are grateful for; with each exhale, think of something you are letting go. For example, you might inhale the feeling of confidence and exhale the feeling of doubt.

1 (8-ounce) Mason jar

3 plastic pipettes

5 drops juniper oil

5 drops lavender oil

3 drops lemon oil

1 cup Himalayan salt (texture can be coarse or fine)

▸ Makes: 1 cup (1 use)

▸ Topical use

▸ Safe for ages 5+

⚠ Do not use for 12 hours before being in direct sunlight or a tanning bed.

1. Using the plastic pipettes, add the essential oils to a small glass bowl and stir to mix them together.

2. Add the Himalayan salt and stir to combine.

3. If you prefer to store this for future use, pour into a Mason jar and label the jar.

4. When you are ready to use it, pour the salt mixture into the bathtub and fill with warm water.

5. Enjoy and soak away the day!

# tension relief bath salt

This bath salt contains the perfect combination of ingredients to relieve tension you accrue throughout the day. Epsom salt works to repair damaged and dry skin, relieve muscle tension and pain, decrease stress levels, and reduce inflammation. Adding progressive muscle relaxation will help immensely. Take a few deep breaths, then mentally scan your body—wherever you are feeling tension, tighten those muscles and hold for 5 to 10 seconds. When you exhale, relax the muscles and feel the tension melt away.

1 (8-ounce) Mason jar

3 plastic pipettes

4 drops ginger oil

5 drops lavender oil

3 drops lemon oil

1 cup Epsom salt (texture can be coarse or fine)

▸ Makes: 1 cup (1 use)

▸ Topical use

▸ Safe for ages 5+

⚠ Do not use for 12 hours before being in direct sunlight or a tanning bed.

1. Using the plastic pipettes, add the essential oils to a small glass bowl and stir to mix them together.

2. Add the Epsom salt and stir to combine.

3. If you prefer to store this for future use, pour into a Mason jar and label the jar.

4. When you are ready to use it, pour the salt mixture into the bathtub and fill with warm water.

5. Enjoy and release the tension!

# deep relax shower steamer

Are you short on time or dislike baths? Showers can be therapeutic, too! As soon as the water hits this shower steamer, the essential oils are released into the steam. Take deep breaths to inhale the aroma and feel your body and mind relax. To make the shower even more therapeutic, lather soap on your body and, as it washes off and goes down the drain, imagine your thoughts, doubts, and fears being washed away.

3 plastic pipettes

40 drops juniper oil

50 drops lavender oil

30 drops vetiver oil

2 cups baking soda

1 cup citric acid

3 to 5 tablespoons water

▸ Makes: about 6 tablets

▸ Indirect inhalation

▸ Safe for ages 5+

1. Using the plastic pipettes, add the essential oils to a small glass bowl. Gently stir the oils for about 1 minute to combine. Set aside.

2. Mix the baking soda and citric acid in a medium glass bowl, stirring until they're combined.

3. Slowly stir the water into the dry ingredients, 1 tablespoon at a time, until the mixture is thick and smooth. Add the essential oils to this mixture and stir until combined.

4. Firmly press the mixture into a silicone mold or muffin tin.

5. Allow the tablets to dry for about 24 hours.

6. Place 1 tablet on the floor of your shower. When the water hits the tablet, it will release the essential oils into the steam. Breathe deeply as you shower until the tablet has dissolved entirely.

7. Enjoy and relax!

# resources

Here are some further resources
for anyone looking to learn more about essential
oils, aromatherapy, diet, and weight loss.

## Aromatherapy

*Essential Oils: A Handbook for Aromatherapy Practice* by Jennifer Peace Rhind. London: Jessica Kingsley Publishers, 2012.

*The Healing Intelligence of Essential Oils* by Kurt Schnaubelt. New York: Healing Arts Press, 2011.

*Medical Aromatherapy: Healing with Essential Oils* by Kurt Schnaubelt. Madison, WI: Frog Books, 1999.

*New York Institute of Aromatic Studies.* www.aromaticstudies.com

*Sage Mind and Body.* www.sagemindandbodymn.com

*375 Essential Oils and Hydrosols* by Jeanne Rose. Berkeley, CA: North Atlantic Books, 1999.

## Guidance

*Bloom for Yourself* by April Green. Detroit, MI: Flower Press Publishing, 2017.

*Earn Your Happy* (podcast).

*Girl, Wash Your Face* by Rachel Hollis. Nashville, TN: Thomas Nelson, 2018.

*Healers Wanted.* www.healerswanted.com

*Insight Timer Meditation* (app).

*Soulful Woman Guidance Cards* by Shushann Movsessian and Gemma Summers. Woodbury, MN: Llewellyn Publications, 2016.

*Spirit Junkie Affirmation* (app).

*The Universe Has Your Back* by Gabrielle Bernstein. Carlsbad, CA: Hay House, 2018.

*You Can Heal Your Life* by Louise L. Hay. Carlsbad, CA: Hay House, 1984.

## Health and Weight Loss

*The Detox Miracle Sourcebook* by Robert Morse. Chino Valley, AZ: Kalindi Press, 2013.

*The Dorito Effect* by Mark Schatzker. New York: Simon & Schuster, 2016.

*Forks Over Knives: The Plant-Based Way to Health* by Gene Stone. New York: The Experiment, 2011.

*Integrative Nutrition.* www.integrativenutrition.com

*Integrative Nutrition: A Whole-Life Approach to Health and Happiness* by Joshua Rosenthal. New York: Integrative Nutrition, Inc., 2018.

## Safety

*Essential Oil Safety* by Robert Tisserand and Rodney Young. London: Churchill Livingstone, 2013.

# index

# acknowledgments

I would like to thank a few people for helping me get to this point in my life.

My chiropractor, Joessa Austin, has been by my side since day one when I knew I needed a change. She helped me change my diet, lose weight, and maintain the results. She also hosted a women's empowerment event that gave me the courage to start health coaching and aromatherapy training, which led to opening my own business—and writing this book!

My acupuncturist, Lacey Cline, worked alongside my chiropractor to support my body through the process. Acupuncture and cupping have helped balance my body, mind, and soul, as well as give my body the strength and recovery to exercise regularly.

Lastly, I am thankful for my family—I wouldn't be the person I am today without them helping me shape my life.

# about the author

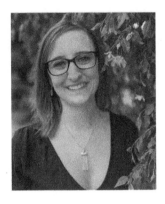

**Samantha Boerner** is incredibly passionate about health and wellness, driven by her own struggles with weight, anxiety, OCD, panic disorder, and insomnia.

She owns Sage Mind and Body in Burnsville, Minnesota, offering custom aromatherapy, signature aromatherapy blends, and health and lifestyle coaching. She holds a NAHA Level 1 Aromatherapy Certification (with Level 2 in process), Integrative Nutrition Health Coach Certification, and a bachelor's degree in Healthcare Administration from Liberty University. These certifications taught Samantha how to help others create and maintain a healthy lifestyle and diet, as well as how to develop customized products that address a range of issues such as digestion, sleep, anxiety, acne, and muscle aches/pains.

Samantha's past work in a chiropractic and mental health office helps her see healthcare from a holistic perspective, and—perhaps most importantly—her personal health journey gives her extensive real-world experience. Through her own struggles, she has tested the efficacy of a variety of methods and products.

Samantha truly loves what she does, and is always eager to help others reach their goals.